THE COMPREHENSIVE HERBALISM GUIDE FOR BEGINNERS

LEARN HOW TO PICK, GROW AND MAKE YOUR OWN HERBAL MEDICINE IN ONLY 3 SIMPLE STEPS

TOM PEACE

Special Offer

As part of the book, it is included a completely FREE Bonus guide that includes simple and surprising hacks and tips to improve your cooking skills. If you want to discover the 7 Fascinating Hacks and Tips for cooking with herbs, click on the link or scan the QR code below.

Link

https://mailchi.mp/a0e0be324cea/7-fascinating-hacks-and-tips-for-cooking-with-herbs

QR Code

CONTENTS

INTRODUCTION

Western medicine is, without a doubt, vital. Numerous severe illnesses necessitate drug-based treatment to remain alive and healthy. Until recently, people were able to lead healthy and balanced lifestyles. However, we know that medicinal herbs cannot heal certain conditions. In such instances, we are forced to employ conventional medicine. So let us look for a cure for everything else in the natural world.

My name is Tom Peace. For me, herbalism is a way of life. By taking regular walks and paying attention to them, we can learn to appreciate the abundance of herbal remedies that surrounds us. While some doctors say that herbs don't work, they are still an excellent way to stay healthy.

My grandma brought me into her garden as a child and educated me about flora. As we went into the woodland, the scent of oak trees filled the air. She applied fresh bay leaves to my skin to protect me from poison oak and keep mosquitoes away. She utilized fresh nettle juice to aid me with the stinging welts after falling into a cluster of nettle plants. Her teachings were concise and straightforward. Her words, like hers, brought tears to my eyes and ached my heart. Due to the enchantment of her garden during my childhood, I continued on my adventure into the green.

It's been a long time since I learned about the medicinal qualities of herbs from some highly knowledgeable individuals. I've visited numerous locations where herbs have been used for centuries, discovered countless other plants, and studied herbal therapy's science and art. My grandmother taught me valuable lessons. These are among the most critical things I've learned throughout my life. I want to educate you on specific concepts that are both basic and critical. Individuals who know about herbs and how they might benefit from them develop a greater appreciation for nature and a more serene way of life.

This is an Herbalist Handbook for Beginners (craft your herbal medicine in just three steps). First, an introduction to herbal medicine is provided in this book. The introduction is followed by three steps to make your natural herbal treatments. The three steps are learning about herbs, planting a garden, and using herbs in natural treatments.

Herbal medicine has grown in popularity significantly during the last few decades. People gradually regain trust in nature and recognize our vital role in the world. Now that we've all met, it's time to get serious about herbal remedies. Herbalism is one of my favorite things to teach since it is versatile and beneficial.

Regular exposure to herbs, like sports, martial arts, music, and the arts, can help you live a longer, healthier life. As a result, those who use herbs regularly have been shown to live longer, healthier lives. This book aims to teach people about herbalism in a fun and educational way.

Typically, we think of aromatic or culinary herbs when we think about herbs. Basil, rosemary, thyme, sage, and peppermint are the most commonly used herbs. While these herbs are delicious when added to cuisine, did you know they may also be used to treat and protect against bites, stings, and headaches? These culinary herbs are perfect for you, but any plant with healing properties is an herb, even if it's just a single flower or a huge tree.

You most likely reside in an area that has not been as developed as suburban areas. There are numerous lovely and beneficial herbs growing all around you, but you may be unaware of them. You should be aware of which plants are helpful to you before searching for berries, leaves, blossoms, and twigs. That is where this book enters the picture.

Herbs that are beneficial to your health can be found in different plants. Certain therapeutic plants like sun or shade might be herbaceous, woody, perennials, or annuals. Numerous plants include therapeutic components in their seeds, bark, roots, leaves, and flowers. The likelihood is that you've been using herbal medicine for an extended period without realising it. Numerous spices and herbs commonly used in cooking have therapeutic effects and are therefore referred to as medicinal herbs. We may use numerous additional things in our kitchens to prepare salves, teas, and poultices.

COVID shutdowns and disruptions over the past two years have taught us that we must be able to care for ourselves and our loved ones. Thinking for ourselves requires us to be inventive and flexible in addressing challenges. For example, COVID-19 estimates that about two billion people lack access to adequate healthcare and medicine. In addition, since the outbreak of the pandemic, there have been reports of countries, companies, and individuals stockpiling medications, further restricting access to the general public. As a result, there has been a rise in fake medicines and questionable health products that haven't been tested or proven safe.

We can no longer rely on international pharmaceutical businesses or governments that restrict (and often block) the free flow of items across borders because of the pandemic and the continued abuse of intellectual property rules. Instead, we must rely on our knowledge and ability to take care of ourselves and our families when unforeseen circumstances like those outlined above impede access to medicine and other health items. So, it's time to turn to herbalism! Thanks to economic and powerful herbal medicines, you will be able to do so, but you will also be able to do so confidently. This book not only teaches you how to use and find high-quality herbs, but it also teaches you how to become more self-sufficient and take charge of your own life and health care.

I've condensed centuries of herbal knowledge into a single, practical volume. With this medicinal herb guide, you'll be able to learn about long-forgotten natural health approaches. This handbook is more comprehensive than any other on the market, meticulously researched, and designed for simplicity of use. It will teach you how to harvest and administer low-cost, do-it-yourself remedies, from planting suggestions to building your natural medicine cabinet, from old procedures to current uses, suitable for beginners and seasoned herbalists alike. In addition, this book provides access to nearly two thousand years of herbal medicine-making history, which may help you save money on prescription medications. This book is an invaluable resource for both professional and amateur herbalists.

So, if you're ready, let's be pioneers in the self-reliant revolution, starting today! I hope that reading this book will start you on an exciting journey that will benefit you for the rest of your life. I hope you find this book precisely what I intended it to be: a helpful guide to the great adventure of herbalism. Today is a fantastic day to study herbalism! The following chapters will teach you a lot more. Are you willing to learn more? Now is the time to start learning and having fun!

STEP ONE: KNOW YOUR HERBS

WHY USE HERBAL MEDICINE?

Herbal Medicine's Many Advantages:

More reasonably priced than traditional medical treatment:

It might cost thousands of dollars a month to see a doctor and buy prescribed medication. Grow your medicinal herbs and use them to manufacture your tinctures at home.

Effective in the treatment of long-term conditions:

Herbal therapies tend to be more successful for long-term chronic sickness than conventional medicine. Changing one's diet and supplementing with herbs can alleviate symptoms of PCOS, arthritis, and chronic fatigue syndrome more than conventional treatment.

Enhances the body's defenses:

The immune system is boosted and strengthened by many plants in herbal medicine since this type of medicine focuses on solving the root of the problem. This, of course, aids in the prevention of a wide range of diseases.

Prescription drugs are more difficult to obtain than herbal remedies:

Herbal medications also have the advantage of being widely available. You can purchase herbs over the counter without a doctor's prescription. It is also possible to grow plants at home. In addition, herbs may be the only therapy option for many people in distant areas.

Herbs can stabilize hormones and metabolism:

Certain plants can regulate hormones. Due to many powerful chemicals in herbs, trying to use just one of these chemicals can often significantly impact the overall benefits of herbal therapy.

Fewer side effects:

Natural therapies are generally well-tolerated and have fewer adverse side effects than synthetic medications. In addition, unlike pharmaceutical treatments, herbs are made of natural components, which may explain why they are less likely to induce side effects.

Synergistic effects:

When herbs are used together, they are more effective. The combined benefits of many different plants are often better than the effects of just one herb.

Increased savings:

Drugs prescribed by a doctor are pricey. Medications made from natural resources, such as herbs, can be produced at a lower cost because of their abundance and accessibility. A reduced cost of production usually translates into a lower price at the point of sale. Herbal cures help patients save money on prescriptions upfront, but they also educate them on managing their health better and provide them with the knowledge and skills they need to be healthy and heal themselves. Using this information, people can improve their health and avoid costly chronic illnesses such as diabetes and heart disease, which result in high medical expenditures, medication costs, and lost wages.

Self-healing:

As a rule, prescription medicines are used to conceal symptoms rather than treat the root cause of the problem. On the other hand, herbal medication may encourage people to pay attention to what their bodies are saying and find the source of their pain or suffering. A patient's health could improve faster if they engage with a doctor specializing in complementary and alternative medicine.

Empowerment:

Taking charge of one's health is a primary motivation for many herbal therapy people. An excellent natural healer teaches people what their bodies require and how to keep them in good condition. It's unlikely that a healer will just offer a prescription to a patient to mask their suffering.

Improved overall health:

There are numerous health advantages to using natural remedies. When it comes to treating sickness, many natural therapies are focused on finding out what's wrong rather than just suppressing symptoms. Rather than relying on drugs, this method is more likely to lead to better health. Herbal therapy is more than just an antidote to disease. Instead, it helps to strengthen the body as a whole. Natural treatments may be more effective than prescription pharmaceuticals in preventing and treating infections among people who prefer to use them instead of relying on Big Pharma.

Finally, the gut is supported by natural medicine. As a result of using herbal medicine, the digestive process is made easier, and the growth of beneficial microorganisms in the gut is promoted.

HARNESS THE
HEALING POWER
OF HERBS

What You Need to Know About Herbal Medicine: Using Plants as Medicine

You'll likely find a wide variety of herbal products on display in a health food store. Herbal medicines are not a new concept. They've been around for a long time. However, thanks to a recent expansion in their availability, people who aren't familiar with their traditional applications can now easily purchase them. Food, tea, and beauty items all contain herbs. In addition, a wide variety of herbal ghees and skin creams are available. But, is there a way to tell which ones are best for you? These details are covered in this chapter for you to use herbs safely, politely, and productively.

Know your needs

Before you start any herbal treatments, make a list of why you want to incorporate herbs into your wellness regimen. Has a specific issue come up that you'd like to get rid of? Some plants are evaluated as safe and moderate enough for general well-being. Therefore, their presence in herbal items and dietary supplements is not uncommon.

Herbs can help with the following conditions:

- Boosting immunity

- Promoting restful sleep.

- Encouraging alertness or a good mood

- Reducing stress

- Antioxidants

In many traditional societies and the United States, herbal remedies for health and well-being are commonplace, and it's relatively easy to build a toolbox of herbs that can support the body, mind, and spirit. In addition, people usually think these herbs are safe to use in small amounts and mild preparations, such as teas, to keep their bodies healthy.

If you want to cure a specific ailment, it's best to seek the advice of a medical practitioner first. A suitable dosage will ensure that it is safe, effective, and tailored to your specific requirements. An herbal formula may be used to achieve the best results by using exact amounts of various herbs in specific proportions. When a single herb is used, the effect can differ depending on how much the person took.

Herbs may be the same for general well-being and specific ailments, but the frequency, quantity, or type of extract may be different. It's crucial to see a doctor if you're dealing with a specific health issue because it can get confusing. All of a patient's symptoms and medical history are considered when prescribing herbal medicines.

Therefore, you should seek the advice of a knowledgeable, certified, and experienced specialist. Your doctor can advise you about probable drug interactions if you take any pharmaceutical drugs. A skilled practitioner can also ensure that your herbs are of the highest quality and aren't contaminated by fillers or other additives.

When buying herbs and other nutritional supplements, customers must keep their expectations realistic. Many herbs and supplements on the internet are not as potent as those a practitioner may prescribe.

Everyone must realize that their health and healing journeys are unique. To discover what makes someone feel their best, it's essential to begin with, the most basic questions. Several herbs may interact with prescribed drugs. Visit your doctor and a certified herbalist to ensure there are no interactions.

Understand the customs

Some herbs have a long history, while others are newer and modern. Traditional herbs may not be found in other traditions. In addition, non-herbal remedies are sometimes used in conjunction with herbal treatments in some cultures. That's why it's critical to conduct thorough research and speak with an expert. The following are just a few instances of traditional medicinal practices that make use of herbs:

•African herbalism and Yorùbá medicine

•Ayurveda

•Chinese traditional medicine

•Western herbal medicine

•Naturopathy

•Indigenous traditional medicine.

There is a possibility that herbs can be misconstrued or mistreated if removed from their traditional setting. They may be overstated or understated. As far as conventional medicine is concerned, practically every culture has its system. There may be a lot of different ways to use herbal medicine.

Ayurveda, for example, is a complete system of ancient medicine that can provide hints to attaining optimal health in a way that we don't generally think about in Western culture. This can have a huge impact when it comes to one's healing!

If you've heard that herbs are helpful for you, you shouldn't take them just because of that. It would be best if you didn't rely on your research when consuming herbs. It's easier to find excellent herbs when you shop online. It is common in many herbal traditions for people to be able to use plants for their own or their family's health. Beyond herbalism, these systems keep essential cultural values, history, traditions, and medical knowledge.

What to look for when buying herbs

The following questions should be on your list when it comes time to buy herbs:

● Is the herb high-grade and potent?

● What steps are involved in the preparation process?

● Is it sourced ethically and sustainably?

● How may the herb be helped or hindered by what you eat, take, or do?

When deciding whether an herb is safe for you, do your research first.

Where do the herbs come from?

It is possible to obtain herbs from several sources. They can be harvested from the wild or raised on a farm. The environment in which herbs are grown, and their strength can be influenced by where they are grown, making sourcing a critical consideration. Herbs thrive best in their native environment. A family environment for herbs is similar to how we feel at home in our own homes. They're recommended to grow alongside other herbs to increase their favorable attributes. It's getting more difficult because herbalism is becoming more commercialized, but experts still prefer to buy their herbs directly from the grower.

In the Ayurveda books, there is a specific procedure for collecting herbs. When it comes to collecting some herbs, you're meant to do so at a particular time and manner. In today's world, that approach is a bit difficult. Experts recommend knowing where your herbs come from to ensure quality and transparency. Learn about the procedures of the firms you're buying from and the products they're selling so that you may support local businesses as much as possible.

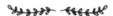

What method is used to prepare the herbs?

It is vital to look at how herbs are made and how to eat them the best way.

Among the herbal preparations are:

- Powders

- Poultices

- Capsules

- Balms and salves

- Infusions

- Tinctures

- Teas and tisanes

There are many ways to preserve herbs, depending on what they're used for and how long you want to keep them. Processed herbs, according to experts, are essential for maintaining potency and making their use more convenient. Herbs have been prepared for millennia and continue to be processed before usage, which is something to keep in mind. For practicality, tradition, and safety reasons, most herbs must be processed before humans may consume them. Medical ghee and oil preserve potency and prevent herbs from being wasted. This method can keep herbs fresh for an additional year. However, the effectiveness of fresh herbs may last only a few days. Taking herbal tinctures is one of the most acceptable ways to absorb herbs because they conserve potency, have a long shelf life, and can boost the herb's usefulness in some situations.

Fresh or dried

Decide if you want fresh or dried herbs before you go shopping. Poultices, tinctures, and teas or tisanes made from fresh herbs are typical. On the other hand, you can consume dried herbs as capsules, beverages, or even just as they are. Experts say there's no one-size-fits-all answer as fresh vs. dried goes. Consumers need to buy in-season herbs if they plan on using or processing them quickly to get the most out of them. Dry herbs are also more convenient and may be enhanced by the drying process.

How potent are these herbs?

You can accurately assess the quality and potency of herbs by relying on reputable experts and conducting your research into the methods used in their preparation, processing, and production. Herbs have a more significant impact than simply eating a healthy diet when used correctly. Even typical culinary spices like black pepper might have this effect because plants that are not cultivated may not be as strong as those grown in their natural setting. To be successful with herbal medicine, you must find the right herb. If the herb you're taking isn't the right one for you, then the issue of potency is moot.

Be cautious about contamination

There is no FDA regulation of herbs and supplements, which means that many herbal products on the market are not evaluated for quality, potency, or contamination. Fillers may also be used to make production more cost-effective.

Contaminants include

●Pollens

●Fungi and molds

●Toxic heavy metals

●Prescription drugs

●Fillers

●Insects

●Rodents

●Toxin

●Pesticides

●Dust

●Parasites

●Microbes

Doing your homework and asking for referrals from trusted practitioners is a wonderful idea. Unfortunately, the supplement industry has had its share of bad actors. As a result, scammers are increasingly peddling items that may contain heavy metals. Because of a lack of regulations, consumers are responsible for conducting their research. One way to ensure that you're getting the best quality herbs is to buy them from a reputable, qualified practitioner. Industry professionals also make suggestions to research manufacturing methods, purchase from organizations that emphasize quality control, and use organic herbs whenever possible. Unfortunately, the FDA does not regulate herbs. If you don't get your herbs from a certified herbalist, you'll have to rely on the label. As a result, the effectiveness and quality of what's inside are largely at the whim of the producer or manufacturer.

Sustainability

Another factor to keep in mind when purchasing herbs is their long-term viability. This encompasses the planet's health, the health of the herb ecosystems, and the health of the many herb species. Wild-harvested herbs may be more effective, but they may also be endangered or over-harvested. The cultivated option may be the best choice in this situation. In this case, too, there are no hard-and-fast rules. What's important is that you do your research and only purchase herbs from practitioners or firms you can trust. In addition, you should use herbs sustainably and ethically. There is no one-size-fits-all approach to the problem of preserving an herb for the long term.

ANTI-INFLAMMATORY HERBS

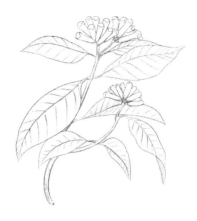

Clove (Syzygium aromaticum)

Overview

A native of Indonesia, the clove (Syzygium aromaticum) is a fragrant evergreen. Dried flower buds have long been used in Ayurvedic and Chinese medicine as spices. They are a common ingredient in meats, sauces, soups, stews, and rice. The chemical eugenol, which is contained in clove oil, may be able to alleviate pain and stop the spread of disease. Cloves are used as both an expectorant and a medicine. Difficulty breathing, diarrhea, and hernias can all be helped with clove oil. It also aids in the alleviation of oral irritation and inflammation. It can also be applied directly to the skin as an anti-irritant.

Health advantages

●Clove oil has been linked to a range of health benefits, including ease of the pain of injections in the mouth. The clove-based gel was found to be as effective as benzocaine in alleviating dental pain (a local anesthetic).

●Our bodies need manganese to keep our brains regular and build strong bones. Cloves abound in manganese, fiber, vitamins, and minerals, making them an excellent source of nutrition.

●People with diabetes or prediabetes may find that clove extract aids in glucose regulation. In healthy adults, clove extract can reduce blood sugar levels.

●It can help make ethanolic clove extract, which can be used in several ways, including as a spot treatment for acne. You can also use clove oil to make ethanolic clove extract.

●Some gram-negative bacteria are inhibited by clove oil.

●Protecting cells from damage that could lead to cancer is the primary function of oxidants. Cloves have a high antioxidant content. Research shows that cloves can slow the growth of several malignancies in humans.

●Scientists have also looked into using cloves as a therapy for obesity. Research has shown that adding clove extract to a high-fat diet can help people stay slim.

• Cloves, which contain a high concentration of antioxidants, may help to protect the liver from harm. Chemicals such as eugenol may reverse cirrhosis in certain patients, which is found in cloves.

• Nigericin and cloves assist in promoting the absorption of glucose from the blood into cells and the creation and functioning of insulin-producing cells. When combined with a healthy diet, cloves may help control blood sugar levels.

• Cloves include compounds beneficial to the body's ability to maintain bone mass. Loss of bone mass can induce osteoporosis, which can lead to fractures. Bone formation benefits from the high manganese content of cloves.

How to use

• You can use ground cloves the same way you would use cinnamon or ginger to flavor baked items like applesauce and oatmeal. Cloves may also be used to make chai, a popular beverage in India and Pakistan that is made with tea, spices, and milk. Depending on the specific recipe, it is possible to utilize cloves in both savory and sweet dishes.

Dosage

•An essential element in many recipes, clove is often found in the form of a garnish. It can be found in many additional items besides mouthwashes, such as gels, lotions, and oils.

Possible Side Effects

•A component of clove oil called eugenol has been shown to have a negative impact on gut flora diversity when taken orally. In general, you should not consume clove oil in large amounts. Swallowing cloves can cause severe burns to the throat. You can apply clove oil to the skin or gums, or it can be used as a mouthwash. Prevent children and newborns from inadvertently consuming clove oil. You should avoid clove products during pregnancy and lactation.

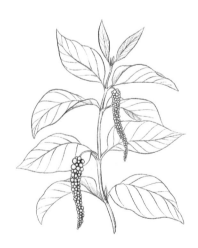

Peppercorn (Piper nigrum)

Overview

Black pepper is a common ingredient in many cuisines around the world. It was known as the "king of spices" in ancient Ayurvedic medicine. To date, pepper has been employed in Ayurveda to treat many different conditions. Menstrual abnormalities and difficulties with the nose, throat, and ears were the most common reasons. Black pepper is grown mainly in tropical Asian countries. Arthritis, asthma, and digestive problems are among the conditions for which black pepper is utilized as a remedy. Applying black pepper extract to the skin can relieve measles, nerve discomfort, and itchy skin, all of which are symptoms of mite-borne illness.

Health advantages

•The combination of black pepper and turmeric is said to be cancer-preventive. You can make a drink by combining turmeric with black pepper. You can ward off cancer and other potentially deadly diseases with the antioxidants and carotenoids found in this drink.

•When consumed raw, black pepper causes the stomach to produce hydrochloric acid. Ingesting hydrochloric acid keeps your intestines in good shape and stops digestive problems from happening.

•The regular addition of pepper to your diet can alleviate the symptoms of constipation.

•People who eat black pepper every day can keep diarrhea and colon cancer at bay.

•Keep your skin's original color by using black pepper to protect it from any form of discoloration. Black pepper can help prevent wrinkles and other skin conditions if taken early in life. Wrinkles and age spots are also kept at bay.

•Because of its anti-inflammatory properties, black pepper is said to help if you have dandruff. Rinse your hair with warm water and a little bit of crushed black pepper after 30 minutes of soaking. Your hair will be shiny and silky after using this remedy.

•Peppercorn may aid weight loss by mixing this secret spice into your green tea. Phytonutrients included in this spice help break down fat. You'll also see an increase in your metabolic rate. This is something you should eat regularly.

•Depression is a prevalent and potentially fatal condition. To lift their spirits, black pepper can be administered to those who are depressed. When you eat raw black pepper, mood-enhancing chemicals enter your brain and keep your thoughts at ease.

●You can treat colds and coughs with black pepper.

●Congestion can be relieved with the use of black pepper and honey. When you breathe in the vapor from hot water flavored with black pepper and eucalyptus oil, you will be able to clear up your chest.

●Pepper's medicinal properties can help ease joint pain caused by arthritic conditions. Gout can also be prevented by taking this herb. Taking this herb can also help alleviate back and joint discomfort. Excessive perspiration and urination aid in the removal of toxins from the body.

Possible Side Effects

●Black pepper is probably safe to eat in the quantities commonly found in food. Consuming too much black pepper can induce stomach trouble and a burning sensation in the mouth and throat. Before you eat black pepper or take supplements, talk to your doctor about how likely your medications will interact with black pepper.

●There are no known harmful effects of using black pepper oil. Pregnant or nursing women can safely apply black pepper to their skin. Black pepper can be taken by mouth in common amounts in most people's diets.

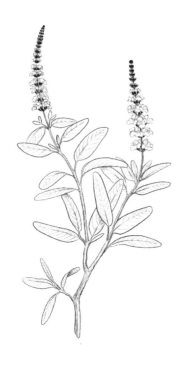

Sage (Salvia officinalis)

Overview

Sage is an aromatic herb, native to the Mediterranean. It belongs to the same family as rosemary, basil, oregano, and thyme, which are also mints. Herb seasonings like sage can be added to stuffing for chicken and pigs, as well as sausages. Sage is widely used in tiny doses because of its earthy scent and flavor. Some species are particularly well-suited for decorative purposes due to the stunning foliage and blooms they produce. Sage can alleviate the chemical imbalances in the brain, which may help those with memory and thinking problems. This condition may also impact insulin and sugar metabolism. Sage is used to curing post-surgical pain, cancer pain, sore throats, and sunburns.

Health advantages

●Sage contains carnosic and rosmarinic acids, which are potent antioxidants. Antioxidants fight both free radicals and inflammation.

●Sage has been around for a long time. It is a purifying plant, both physically and morally. Sage is a popular ingredient in many cuisines because of its antibacterial and fragrant characteristics.

●Sage essential oil can also be used to get rid of body odor and treat wounds and skin infections caused by bacteria called staphylococcus, which can cause infections.

●The healing properties of this herb can also help with memory improvement.

●Sage extracts may help people with mild to severe Alzheimer's.

●Sage may help with digestive difficulties. In some cases, diarrhea might be relieved by taking the sage extract.

●Sage may also be beneficial to the health of women. Sage is an herbal remedy for menopausal hot flashes. Anecdotal evidence suggests that sage can help new mothers who are trying to wean themselves off breastfeeding or produce too much milk.

•Taking common sage (Salvia officinalis) three times a day for two months may help people with high cholesterol. It may also help people with high cholesterol.

Dosage

•Sage is an active ingredient in gel caps, oral extracts, capsules, topical lotions, and ointments. Even though there isn't a set dosage recommendation, most people can safely consume up to 1,000 mg per day. Sage creams should be used as directed by the manufacturer.

Possible Side Effects

•Thujone, the neurotoxin responsible for absinthe's mind-altering effects, may be found in sage. Sage can induce life-threatening adverse effects, including vomiting, dizziness, rapid heart rate, tremors, seizures, and kidney damage if swallowed in large doses. People who have diabetes may have dangerously low blood sugar levels if they overuse sage.

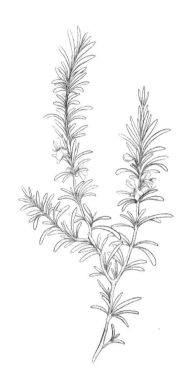

Rosemary (Salvia rosmarinus)

Overview

Many cuisines worldwide rely on rosemary as an essential herb, which is native to the Mediterranean region. Since ancient times, it has been lauded for its medicinal powers. A range of diseases, including muscle pain, memory loss, and a compromised immune system, have long been treated with rosemary. Many people prefer rosemary because of its flavor, aroma, and health benefits. Modern scientific research has supported the long-held belief that rosemary is a potent therapeutic herb. You can make infused oils and teas from the leaves of this plant. Many people use rosemary as a natural cure for a wide range of problems, including memory loss, dyspepsia, and fatigue.

Health advantages

●Rosemary oil has a lot of health benefits when it comes to relieving gas, bloating, and constipation in the digestive tract. Additional benefits include an increase in appetite and control over the formation of bile. Use five drops of rosemary essential oil and one teaspoon of almond or coconut oil to massage your stomach to alleviate gas and bloating. Regular usage of rosemary oil helps cleanse the liver and increase the gallbladder's ability to function correctly.

●The aroma of rosemary essential oil has reduced the stress hormone cortisol. When you're in "fight-or-flight" mode, your cortisol levels increase. Chronic stress manifests as weight gain, oxidative damage, and hypertension. Stress can be quickly relieved with the use of rosemary essential oil. Spraying it on your pillow at night may help you relax.

●Massage the affected region with rosemary oil to relieve pain and reduce inflammation. You can use it to relieve pain from sprains, strains, arthritis, and headaches. Take a hot bath with a few drops of rosemary oil.

●Cold, flu, and allergy congestion can be relieved using rosemary oil. Respiratory problems may benefit from the scent's antibacterial characteristics. In addition, its antispasmodic properties may be beneficial in the treatment of bronchitis.

●Apply a few drops of rosemary oil to your hair to keep it looking its best. It aids in the maintenance of healthy, lustrous hair. In addition, a massage with rosemary essential oil can speed up hair growth.

Possible Side Effects

●Keep rosemary out of the reach of children under 18 years. Never eat more than 4 to 6 grams of dry rosemary per day to avoid becoming poisoned. The oil of rosemary, too, should not be taken internally.

●Rosemary can cause miscarriage in pregnant women, so they should not take in a lot of the herb.

●Do not eat rosemary if you have high blood pressure, ulcers, Crohn's disease, or gastrointestinal problems. When consumed in large doses, rosemary leaves can cause nausea and spasms.

●Aspirin and warfarin (blood thinners) may be influenced by rosemary's ability to dilute the bloodstream. In the case of high blood pressure, taking ACE inhibitors may be influenced by the plant. There is a chance that rosemary could make your blood sugar levels go up or down if you take diabetes medicine.

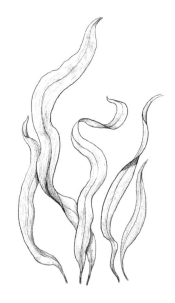

Photo credit: healthline

Spirulina (Spirulina)

Overview

B vitamins and vitamin E are only a few of the elements in spirulina, a blue-green algae powerhouse rich in health-promoting characteristics. This alga can be used as a supplement or a meal. Spirulina, a great source of plant-based protein, has been linked to many health benefits. It is one of the planet's oldest living organisms. It's high in minerals and antioxidants, which may improve your overall health and well-being, both physically and mentally.

Blending it with other foods can mask the bitterness of spirulina like smoothies, yogurt, and juices. Spirulina powder is available in health food stores as a dietary supplement. Spirulina's high protein and vitamin content make it ideal for vegetarians and vegans. In addition, it's thought that spirulina has anti-inflammatory and antioxidant properties and that it can also help the body's immune system be more stable, according to some research.

Health advantages

•Spirulina contains all of the amino acids essential for human well-being. One tablespoon of spirulina has seven grams of protein.

•Spirulina is a good provider of vitamin B12, unlike the vast majority of plant foods.

•Vitamin B12 is vital for the production of energy as well as for the normal functioning of the brain. One tablespoon of spirulina contains 250 percent of your daily vitamin B12 requirement.

•A significant amount of beta-carotene, found in high concentrations in spirulina, is advantageous to the retina. Carotenoids and potent antioxidants are also included in spirulina, which helps fight off free radicals.

•As an effective anti-inflammatory, phycocyanin shields the immune system against the damaging effects of the medicine. There is a lot of phycocyanin in this light green powder.

•Spirulina contains a lot of fiber. Adding additional fiber to your diet may improve your overall health, digestive health, and blood sugar levels. Spirulina can improve your digestive system if you incorporate it into your regular diet.

•A high-folate diet may reduce depression, heart disease, and cancer. One tablespoon of spirulina provides 110% of your daily vitamin B12 requirements.

•The body's vital functions can be supported by consuming enough iron in your diet. Iron aids the immune system, digestion, and overall health. A single tablespoon of spirulina contains 30% of your daily iron requirements.

•Additionally, vitamin A is essential in maintaining a healthy body and mind. Deficiency in vitamin A can lead to bone loss, immune system dysfunction, and cancer risk. About 9000% of the RDA for vitamin A is found in one cup of spirulina.

●Half of the daily required amount of vitamin K is found in one tablespoon of spirulina. You can improve bone health and wound healing by ensuring that your vitamin K levels are sufficient.

●Spirulina has a wide variety of B vitamins. Your body's ability to create enough vitamin B is critical to the health of your cells. Red blood cell formation, energy, and cognitive function improve when you consume this alga. This herb has some beneficial effects on the digestive system, appetite, and nervous system.

●Inflammation can be reduced by GLA, which is found in spirulina (gamma-linolenic acid). Certain naturopathic doctors prescribe GLA supplements to improve insulin sensitivity and aid in weight loss. This medication can also help lessen discomfort symptoms and blood pressure caused by hormones.

●Scientists have discovered anti-inflammatory effects in the omega-3 fatty acids in spirulina. Taking this particular omega-3 may improve heart health, cognitive function, and diabetes management.

●One tablespoon of spirulina has the same amount of calcium as three glasses of milk. Calcium is essential for the health of your bones, muscles, and nervous system.

•Spirulina has a high chlorophyll concentration, making it good detoxifying food. Wheatgrass contains the same amount of chlorophyll as a tablespoon of spirulina.

Dosage

•Spirulina capsules and pills are convenient ways to acquire the daily recommended amount of this alga in your system. Spirulina supplements are normally taken one to three times a day.

•Cumin, lemon juice, and cayenne pepper can all be used to enhance the flavor of spirulina.

Possible Side Effects

•As with any supplement, spirulina has the potential to cause sleepiness, headaches, muscle pain, and sweat. Spirulina can cause an allergic reaction in people sensitive to seaweed, shellfish, or other sea vegetables.

•To avoid activating the immune system, spirulina should be avoided by people with autoimmune illnesses like MS, RA, or Lupus.

•Cellcept, Enbrel, and Humira (adalimumab) are immunosuppressive drugs. You should not take spirulina if you are taking these drugs.

●People who have phenylketonuria, which means they can't digest a certain amino acid, should stay away from spirulina.

●Spirulina has not been tested for safety in pregnant or nursing women. See your doctor before taking spirulina if you are pregnant, nursing, or wanting to get pregnant.

DIGESTIVE HERBS

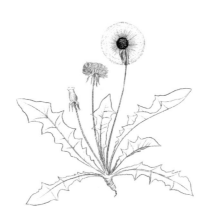

Dandelion root (Taraxacum officinale)

Overview

Native Americans and traditional Chinese medicine have long used the dandelion root to treat stomach and liver problems. Taraxacum officinale, the most common variety of this plant, may be found worldwide. The roots and blooms of the dandelion plant, as well as the leaves, are all edible. It is often used in herbal medicine because of its chicory-like flavor. The root of the dandelion can be roasted and used to make a caffeine-free tea. Compounds in the supplement may help reduce edema, increase urine production, and prevent the formation of crystals in the urine, all of which may contribute to infections of the kidneys and urinary tract. Also, herbal tea and supplements are utilized to improve the skin, liver, and heart health and promote blood glucose management.

Health advantages

●It contains beta-carotene, an antioxidant that shields cells from oxidative stress. According to research, antioxidants like beta-carotene, which are carotenoid antioxidants, are vital for reducing cellular damage. Polyphenols, another form of antioxidant, are also found in abundance.

●In adults, dandelion's bioactive components may help decrease cholesterol levels. In rats fed a high-cholesterol diet, root and leaf extracts from dandelion reduced cholesterol levels.

•In some studies, experts found that dandelions have chemicals that may help keep blood sugar levels in check.

•Dandelions could be used to treat type 2 diabetes because they are antioxidants, fight inflammation, and lower blood sugar.

•Several studies have shown that extracts and compounds from dandelion can help stop inflammation in the body's tissues.

•Dandelions are a rich source of potassium. Clinical research has indicated that potassium can reduce blood pressure.

•Several researchers have proposed dandelion as a weight loss aid. This claim is based on the plant's ability to enhance glucose metabolism and reduce fat absorption. A study suggests that chlorogenic acid, found in dandelions, may help stop people from gaining weight and keeping fat in their bodies.

•According to some studies, dandelions may be able to inhibit the growth of several types of cancer. In experiments, researchers found dandelions to reduce the growth of pancreatic, colon, and liver tumors.

•Research shows that dandelions may help enhance the body's defenses against disease. Dandelions have antiviral and antibacterial properties that scientists have identified.

According to research published in 2014, dandelion seeds have been shown to protect against hepatitis B.

•Dandelion tea is a classic home remedy for relieving constipation and other digestive issues.

•Certain research suggests that the skin may be protected from UV damage by dandelions. The skin is damaged, and the aging process is accelerated by exposure to ultraviolet (UV) light. In a 2015 study on skin cells cultured in a test tube, dandelion was discovered to lower one type of UV light.

Dosage

•Wild dandelions are often eaten raw or cooked, including the leaves, stems, and blossoms. The dried, crushed root is commonly used as a tea or coffee replacement. Dandelion extract, pills, and tinctures are all dandelion-based supplements. The following dosages are indicated for different dandelion types.

○Fresh leaves: 4–10 grams daily.

○Leaf tincture: 0.4–1 teaspoon (2–5 mL) thrice daily.

○2–8 grams of fresh roots per day

○4–10 grams of dried leaves per day

○Dried powder: 250–1,000 mg four times per day.

○Fresh leaf juice: 1 teaspoon (5 mL) twice daily.

○1–2 teaspoons (5–10 mL) of fluid extract daily

Possible side effects

●Wild dandelions are often eaten raw or cooked, including the leaves, stems, and blossoms. The dried, crushed root is commonly used as a tea or coffee replacement. Dandelion extract, pills, and tinctures are all dandelion-based supplements. The following dosages are indicated for different dandelion types:

○Heartburn

○Diarrhea

○A distressed stomach

○Skin inflammation

●Hives, watery eyes, and other symptoms are common in those allergic to dandelion roots. Because of its chemicals, you should not eat dandelion if you are allergic to iodine or latex.

●Pregnant, lactating or breastfeeding women should avoid utilizing dandelion remedies due to the absence of long-term safety research. Dandelion consumption has also been linked to reduced fertility and testosterone levels in women and men, so caution should be exercised when using this herb.

Dandelion plants are likely safe for the vast majority of people, especially when they're consumed in the form of food.

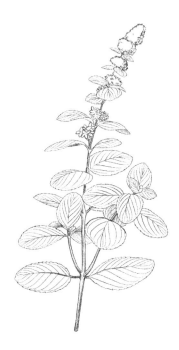

Peppermint (Mentha piperita)

Overview

Peppermint, a fragrant herb in the mint family, is produced through the cross-pollination of water mint and spearmint. The peppermint plant has been treasured as a perennial herb since ancient times. Minty in flavor and soothing nature, it has been used medicinally for generations. As long ago as

1000 BC, researchers found dried peppermint leaves in the pyramids of ancient Egypt. Mints were used as medicine by the Greeks, Romans, and Egyptians. All of the essential oils in peppermint are present in the leaves. It wasn't until the 17th century that a subspecies of peppermint was discovered. Peppermint has been used for medicine for thousands of years, as well as in cooking and beauty products.

Health advantages

•Some studies have suggested that peppermint and other herbal medications can help alleviate children's stomachaches. Several studies have shown that it can help make chemotherapy patients feel less sick and less likely to throw up.

•Irritable bowel syndrome can cause gas, stomach pain, constipation, and diarrhea. Coated peppermint oil capsules may help with these problems.

•Peppermint's primary ingredient is menthol. These substances help alleviate migraine headaches' symptoms, such as sensitivity to light, nausea, and vomiting. You can also eliminate tension headaches by putting a peppermint oil solution on your forehead and temples.

•Peppermint's antibacterial properties may also help eliminate the germs that cause bad breath, making the experience more pleasant.

●Peppermint's antibacterial qualities may help alleviate the symptoms of a common cold or sinus infection. Using menthol can also make it easier to breathe.

●To help you stay alert during the day, peppermint oil may be beneficial. The smell of peppermint oil may help you sleep better at night if you inhale it.

●Peppermint's menthol component might minimize or even eliminate period pain for some people.

●Scientists tested peppermint oil against Listeria, Salmonella, and other pathogens. This chemical was shown to have the ability to halt all three of them.

●Researchers believe peppermint oil may reduce hunger pangs. Weighing less due to this could help you lose some weight.

●During allergy season, peppermint can enhance your outdoor enjoyment. It has Rosmarinus acid, which lowers the body's histamine reaction.

●Peppermint oil capsules have been discovered to assist people in working through difficulties for more extended periods of time without becoming mentally fatigued. This herb's potent aroma may also aid with memory recall and attention span maintenance.

Dosage

•Tea, tablets, and peppermint extracts are all options for obtaining peppermint leaves. You can purchase the oil of peppermint in capsules and beverages. It can be rubbed into the skin or swallowed whole. Because it's so concentrated, only a few drops at a time are necessary. Taking too much oil at one time might be dangerous.

Possible Side Effects

•People sensitive to smoke inhalation may have vomiting and diarrhea due to peppermint use; this is especially true for toddlers under the age of two.

•Peppermint at mealtime can reduce the risk of harm to pregnant women and nursing mothers. There is insufficient evidence to support greater doses as a medical treatment. Pregnant or nursing women should avoid taking higher doses of this medication.

•People with GERD, HNI, arrhythmia or hemolytic anemia should not use peppermint. The same goes for people with gastric reflux disease.

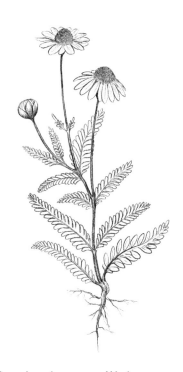

Chamomile (Matricaria chamomilla)

Overview

The Asteraceae family includes chamomile, which is classified as a flowering plant. It has spread worldwide since its inception in Europe and Western Asia. The herb's faint apple scent may have inspired the herb's name (derived from the Greek word chamomile). Studies have shown encouraging outcomes for chamomile tea for various diseases, including cancer and diabetes. As an alternative to black or green tea, chamomile has a mellow, earthy flavor and is a wonderful choice for pregnant women concerned about caffeine. In addition, cancer and cardiovascular disease may be less likely to occur if you consume a diet rich in antioxidants such as spinach. The tea's relaxing and digestion-enhancing properties are two more reasons to try it.

Health advantages

•Several studies have shown that chamomile tea is an effective preventative strategy and a cure-all for several ailments. It also has a soothing impact on the nervous system, making it easier to fall asleep. Antibacterial and immune-boosting qualities are found in this herb.

•Is your nose running with a bad case of sniffles? That's a significant benefit of chamomile. Chamomile tea is an excellent remedy for insomnia, so you may want to check it out. Breathing in the steam from chamomile tea can help with stuffy noses, runny noses, and sore throats.

•Chamomile tea is known for its anti-inflammatory and analgesic properties. Because it relaxes the uterus and cuts down on the production of prostaglandins, it helps alleviate pain.

•The calming properties of chamomile tea have been utilized for gas and indigestion as well as diarrhea and anorexia.

•Chamomile tea was used by the ancient Egyptians, Greeks, and Romans to treat wounds and promote healing. Chamomile (Matricaria chamomilla) is the plant used to make chamomile tea. This plant has anti-inflammatory and anti-microbial properties, which is why it is widely used. You can also use it to treat psoriasis and eczema.

●You can ease stress and depression by drinking tea made from the flowers of the chamomile plant.

●A cup of hot chamomile tea may be beneficial to your skin! This miraculous cure works wonders on the skin because it's a natural bleach. You can improve the health of your skin by drinking chamomile tea. This product gives the skin a healthy, glowing radiance.

●Additionally, chamomile tea may help you get rid of your recurrent breakouts. You can use chamomile tea's anti-inflammatory and antibacterial properties on the skin to reduce spots, get rid of acne scars, and stop new ones from forming.

●Chamomile tea is a beautiful alternative for those with sensitive skin, as it has antioxidants that protect the skin from free radical damage. It helps to reduce the appearance of fine lines and wrinkles and speed up the regeneration of skin cells and tissues.

●Damage from the sun's harmful ultraviolet (UV) rays can cause various skin disorders. A cloth soaked in tea can be applied to a sunburned region after the tea has been brewed and cooled.

Possible Side Effects

Chamomile should be avoided unless prescribed by a doctor for the following people:

•People allergic to pollen may have an allergic reaction to chamomile because it may have pollen from other plants.

•It is suggested that people who have had a bad reaction to chamomile products in the past don't use them again.

•Pediatricians often advise against giving honey and chamomile products to infants and young children.

•Using chamomile as a substitute for a well-established medical treatment is not good. Check with your doctor if drinking chamomile tea could have an adverse effect on any medications you already take.

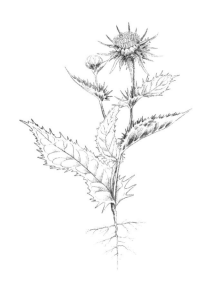

Milk thistle (Silybum marianum)

Overview

This plant is also known as Mary thistle and Holy thistle. Milk thistle leaves are named for the white veins that run through their thick, prickly leaves. If you believe in mythology, you may be able to identify this thorny plant by its purple flowers and white veins. In addition, milk thistles may have some therapeutic properties. Silymarin, a chemical family in the seeds, is thought to have anti-inflammatory and antioxidant qualities. Antioxidant Silymarin is found in the plant's sap and seeds. Antioxidants shield cells from free radical damage. Milk thistle is available in various dosage forms, including capsules and pills, in addition to the liquid extract.

Health advantages

●When your liver breaks down hazardous chemicals, free radicals are generated. Milk thistle may help prevent liver damage by protecting against free radicals.

●It has been shown that milk thistle protects neurons against oxidative damage. This supplement reduces amyloid plaques in Alzheimer's disease rats.

●Milk thistle has been shown to increase bone mineralization, which may help prevent bone loss. Even though no human tests have been done yet, this treatment may help postmenopausal women who are worried about bone loss.

●The use of milk thistle may help alleviate some of the unpleasant effects of some cancer treatments. More research must be done to determine if Silymarin works before it can be given to people with cancer.

●Breastfeeding mothers who took milk thistle had an increase in milk output. This supplement increases prolactin, a hormone that promotes milk production. According to one study, more milk was produced by silymarin-tainted moms than those who took a placebo over six months.

●Acne is caused by skin inflammation. There are no long-term health effects, but they can leave scars. People who took Silymarin for eight weeks saw a 53% decrease in the number of lesions on their skin. Acne sufferers may find milk thistle to be an effective supplement.

•Blood sugar and insulin levels can be improved and even reduced by milk thistle's active components. Milk thistle may help prevent complications from diabetes, such as kidney disease because it is an antioxidant and an anti-inflammatory.

Dosage

•There are no clear guidelines for the proper usage of milk thistle. In addition to the more traditional preparations, you can also take milk thistle as pills, capsules, tea bags, or oral medicines. The dose range is between 175 and 1,000 milligrams. Higher doses are more likely to cause side effects in general.

•Barbero tablets and Iberogast drops treat diabetes and dyspepsia, respectively. Milk thistle dosages of 10 mg and 210 mg have been shown to be effective in clinical trials. Higher doses do not always produce more significant results. Many health food stores, pharmacies, and shops specializing in herbal cures carry milk thistle-containing dietary supplement products. In addition, you can purchase supplements for milk thistle online.

Possible Side Effects

•In general, milk thistle is regarded as safe to ingest.

●In studies, only 1% of the people who got high doses over a long period had bad effects.

●Diarrhea, nausea, and bloating are milk thistle's most prevalent side effects.

●You should proceed with caution if you are allergic to milk thistle. The following are only a few examples:

○Pregnant women shouldn't take this supplement until there is evidence to the contrary.

○If you're allergic to plants in the Asteraceae family, milk thistle could be a problem.

○Due to its ability to lower blood sugar levels, milk thistle has the potential to cause low blood sugar in people with diabetes.

○When milk thistle is used in large doses, it may exacerbate hormone-sensitive conditions, such as breast cancer.

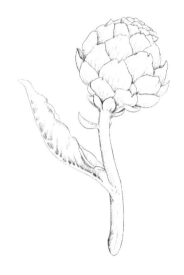

Artichoke (Cynara cardunculus scolymus)

Overview

As a member of the thistle family, artichokes are an excellent source of vitamin A. People in the Mediterranean region have relied on this herb for its medicinal properties for centuries. It's a terrific accompaniment to soups and salads. The leaves, stems, and roots of the plant are used to make therapeutic products. You can treat acid reflux and liver problems with artichoke leaves. It helps with nausea, vomiting, and bloating. In addition to lowering cholesterol, these chemicals also help to protect the liver. Dyspepsia and high cholesterol or other fat levels are among the many conditions for which artichoke is prescribed. You can also treat hepatitis C and IBS with it. Because it has a lot of plant parts, artichoke extract is becoming increasingly popular as a dietary supplement.

Health advantages

•Artichokes rank in the top ten vegetables in terms of ORAC value as an excellent source of antioxidants. Antioxidants and phytonutrients like Cynarin and rutin are abundant in artichokes and the flavonoids quercetin and gallic acid. You can prevent tumors from spreading by eating artichokes. Antioxidants found in artichokes slow the spread of cancerous cells.

•Eating artichokes or artichoke extract has been associated with lowering dangerous cholesterol levels, boosting blood flow, and relieving inflammation. In addition, Cynarin, a potent chemical found in artichokes, has been shown to reduce cholesterol levels naturally.

•Artichokes contain the flavonoid silymarin, which protects the liver. In addition, the fiber and anti-inflammatory properties of the artichoke are thought to help people with IBS and other digestive problems.

•Because of their high fiber content, artichokes are beneficial for various bodily functions. Eating a high-fiber diet can help with both constipation and diarrhea. Fiber aids digestion and makes us feel full after eating because it allows the liver to break down food and remove toxins from the body. In addition to lowering blood pressure and decreasing the risk of heart attack, stroke, and hypertension, fiber provides a slew of additional health benefits. Artichokes are a good source of potassium, which may lower blood pressure.

● It's been shown that eating artichokes boosts insulin sensitivity and production. This is because artichoke fibers reduce the glucose absorption rate into the bloodstream.

● The iron in one cup of artichokes is adequate to provide 10% of the average person's daily iron needs. By eating foods high in iron, you can avoid anemia and other signs of not getting enough iron.

● It is crucial to include antioxidants in your daily diet to avoid wrinkles or skin degradation. In addition, skin wounds, burns, and exposure to common contaminants can benefit from ingesting artichokes.

● Artichoke leaf extract may help treat the symptoms of inflammatory bowel syndrome (IBS), lowering the risk of gastrointestinal illness, diabetes, and obesity. This is because they have prebiotic fibers that help good bacteria grow in your digestive tract.

Dosage

Artichoke extract has been shown to have few known side effects. However, one or more of the following dangers may arise:

•People who are allergic to artichokes or artichoke extract should avoid them.

•Artichoke extract shouldn't be used by pregnant women or nursing because there isn't enough research on how safe it is.

•Since artichokes and artichoke extract can help move bile, people with gallstones or a blocked bile duct should stay away from them.

•In human trials, three doses of 300–640 mg of artichoke leaf extract per day have been found to be the most effective.

•Your doctor can help you determine whether or not artichoke extract is good for you.

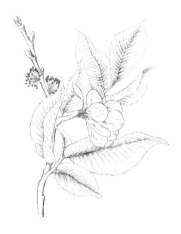

Slippery Elm (Ulmus rubra)

Overview

The slippery elm is a tree native to North America. Traditional Native American medicine uses the inner bark to treat wounds and stomach issues. In traditional Native American medicine, slithering elm was used to cure burns, blisters, ulcers, and skin irritation. You can use water to remove the mucous-like mucilage from its bark. It has been used as a natural remedy in the United States since immemorial. Taken orally, it alleviated symptoms such as coughs, throat irritation, diarrhea, and other digestive issues. This herb is used to treat everything from stomach problems to stress and anxiety.

Health advantages

•Crohn's disease, ulcerative colitis, IBS, and diverticulitis can all benefit from using slippery elm. GERD, heartburn, and laryngitis have all been demonstrated to benefit from the usage of slippery elm, and You can also use it to treat sore throats and laryngitis. You can use sore throat teas and tablets to ease sore throats and other symptoms of the common cold.

•Stiff elm is a traditional remedy for bladder and urinary tract infections.

•Anxiety and stress can be relieved with the gut-healing properties of slippery elm. This is because our mental health is strongly linked to our digestive system. As well as having plant phenolic compounds, slippery elm has a positive effect on both physical and mental health.

•One study found that slippery elm water reduced the intensity of psoriasis symptoms in subjects.

•Women with breast cancer increasingly turn to herbal therapies, including slippery elm. Essiac, which contains slippery elm bark, Indian rhubarb, and sheep sorrel, is frequently prescribed as a breast cancer supplement. According to research, Essiac may have antioxidant and anti-cancer qualities, and one study found that many women felt better after taking the supplement.

Dosage

●Inner bark powder is used as a medicinal ingredient. To make tea, combine two tablespoons of powder and two cups of hot water. Let it steep for two minutes. Preparation of a poultice with a coarse powder and hot water is required (to be applied topically). Use it as a poultice on the affected area. Before taking any supplements, check with your doctor and read the label carefully.

Possible Side Effects

●It hasn't been proven to be harmful or hazardous.

●Slippery bark Slippery elm, primarily composed of mucus, may restrict the amount of medicine your body can absorb. It is recommended that slippery elm bark be taken at least one hour after ingesting another oral medication.

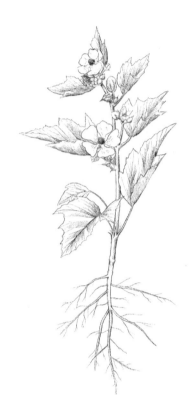

Marshmallow (Althaea officinalis)

Overview

Known as marshmallow root, Althaea Officinalis is a plant that has been used in herbal medicine for centuries. It has been used for centuries to treat gastrointestinal, respiratory, and skin ailments. Its medicinal benefits are mainly due to the presence of mucilage. People turn to marshmallow root for various ailments, including coughs and skin irritations. It comes in powder, tablet, tea, and cough syrup varieties.

Marshmallows are sometimes used as a barrier between the epidermis and the digestive tract. It may also help with cough suppression and infection resistance due to chemicals in it. To be clear, marshmallows are not mallow (Malva sylvestris).

Health advantages

●The antitussive and mucilaginous properties of marshmallow root aid in relieving sore throats and swelling of the lymph nodes. The symptoms of a sore throat, cough, and other respiratory ailments can be relieved. Marshmallow tea is a fantastic cure for pain relief.

●The root's antioxidants, which have been demonstrated to be particularly efficient in the lungs, may prevent cancerous tumor growth. Its high quantities of vitamin C also aid in removing mucus from the lungs, where they are most effective. As a cancer-fighting supplement, the root's vitamin C may strengthen the body's defenses.

●Marshmallow root has been shown in some studies to benefit the respiratory system.

●Due to its high mucilage content, it reduces inflammation of the lining of the digestive tract and the healing of ulcers. Adding a barrier to the digestive tract, Marshmallows can help leaky gut syndrome.

●People with ulcerative colitis or Crohn's disease may benefit from marshmallow roots.

•Marshmallow roots help relieve any infection's swelling, tenderness and burning. When eaten, marshmallow root has been shown to help eliminate bacteria that can cause infections in the urinary tract.

•Interstitial cystitis, a bladder condition, may benefit from marshmallow roots, according to specific sources. If you have a bacterial illness, marshmallow roots and tea from them might help relieve some of your symptoms.

•Marshmallow root's anti-inflammatory characteristics may aid in improving cardiovascular health, as inflammation significantly contributes to cardiovascular disease. In certain studies, marshmallow root has been found to affect cholesterol levels positively.

•Marshmallow root may help treat heartburn, acid reflux, diarrhea, and constipation. It prevents burning by protecting the stomach's inner lining.

•Marshmallow root calms the skin's nervous system, reducing skin inflammation. The root can be applied externally to treat wounds, burns, bug bites, and dry and peeling skin. Because of its mucilage properties, it soothes the skin.

•Additionally, the anti-inflammatory properties of marshmallow root can help treat eczema. The mucilage in marshmallow root may be benefitial for your hair.

Dosage

- You can buy marshmallows in many different forms, like roots, leaves, macerate (which has been soaked in liquid), syrup, and tablets.

- Traditional tea recipes call for dried marshmallow plant parts.

- Another option is to apply marshmallow extract topically to the skin.

- In the past, dosages of 2 to 15 grams daily have been used to alleviate coughs and throat pain.

Possible Side Effects

- Nausea and dizziness may result. A steady increase in dosage can help keep side effects to a minimum by starting with a lower dose and gradually increasing it.

- Drinking an 8-ounce glass of water along with your marshmallow root may help lessen any adverse effects.

- A maximum of four weeks is recommended to experience effects when using this root. Give yourself a week off before starting back up again with the medication.

- Irritation of the skin may result with topical use of marshmallow root. It would be best if you always did patch testing before releasing a complete application.

●Before taking marshmallow root, consult your doctor because it has been linked to lithium and diabetes medications. Also, it can build up in the intestines, making it hard for other medicines to absorb.

You should avoid it if

●If you are pregnant or breastfeeding,

●I have diabetes

●Having surgery in the next two weeks.

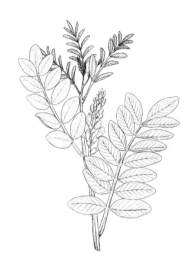

Licorice Root (Glycyrrhiza glabra)

Overview

Liqueur root has long been used as a herbal treatment, derived from the licorice plant's rootstock. Licorice has been used for centuries to treat and flavor food and medication. In Eastern and Western medicine, licorice root has long been utilized as a medicinal herb. The Middle East and Asia are the origins of the plant. Some traditional doctors believe that licorice root can aid with various ailments, including eczema, indigestion, gastritis, and menstrual cramps, to name a few. Because of its chemical composition, licorice is thought to offer anti-inflammatory, anti-cough, and ulcer-healing qualities. In addition, licorice can help with various diseases, including psoriasis, liver enlargement, and canker sores.

Health advantages

•Licorice root has been used in traditional medicine to cure many ailments, including gastric reflux, hot flashes, coughing, and infections caused by bacteria and viruses.

•More than 300 compounds in licorice root give it antibacterial, anti-inflammatory, and antiviral qualities. Aside from acne and eczema, it can treat many other skin disorders. In a two-week study, 60 people with eczema were completely cured by a gel made with licorice root extract.

•Licorice root extract, often available in over-the-counter drugs, can treat symptoms of acid reflux, an upset stomach, and indigestion.

•Peptic ulcers may benefit from licorice root extract, which contains the active ingredient glycyrrhizin. In one study, researchers found that licorice extract was better than omeprazole at preventing these ulcers.

•According to research, cancer cell growth is inhibited or stopped by licorice root extract.

•Some researchers say that licorice root extract and tea could help people with breathing problems.

Dosage

At health food stores and online, there are many licorice root products to choose from. The following are examples of this type of thing:

●Chewable pills

●capsules

●Extracts

●Teas

●Lozenges

●Tinctures

●Powders

There is no right or wrong way to prepare or consume licorice root. However, dosages of 5 to 15 grams per day are safe for short-term use.

Possible Side Effects

●Licorice root is considered safe for short-term use as a supplement or tea, but prolonged use can have significant adverse effects. When the body has excess glycyrrhetinic acid, the stress hormone cortisol can become dangerously high in the bloodstream. It is not recommended that licorice root be consumed by infants, pregnant women, or breastfeeding women. Symptoms of licorice poisoning include congestive cardiomyopathy, pulmonary embolism, and coma.

Potential drug interactions

•Drugs that lower potassium

•Diuretics

•Medication for irregular heartbeat

•Blood thinners

•Blood pressure medications

•Hormone therapy, estrogen, and birth control pills

•Corticosteroids

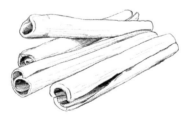

Cinnamon (Cinnamomum)

Overview

From 2000 BC until today, cinnamon has been a popular ingredient in Egyptian cuisine. Sneezing and rheumatism were the diseases practitioners used to treat in the

Middle Age. Cinnamon has traditionally been used to treat respiratory and digestive problems in Ayurvedic medicine. The Egyptians used cinnamon as a perfume, while the Romans used it to mask the stench of burning flesh in funeral pyres. Cinnamon is mentioned numerous times in the Bible as a component of linens, garments, and anointing oil. The two most prevalent types of cinnamon are Ceylon cinnamon and Cassia cinnamon. Both types have different nutritional profiles. Anti-inflammatory, anti-diabetic, antioxidant, and antibacterial ingredients are all found in cinnamon.

Health advantages

•You may improve the management of type 2 diabetes significantly if cinnamon is used daily. Cinnamon contains compounds that mimic insulin's effects, making it beneficial for those with diabetes.

•Cinnamon may be an excellent way to lower your bad cholesterol and raise your good cholesterol simultaneously.

•When it comes to preventing acne-causing microorganisms from spreading, cinnamon can help.

•When combined with cinnamon, cinnamaldehyde has anti-inflammatory and anti-platelet-clumping effects. It can stop inflammation and cells from growing in the wrong way, making it less likely that someone will get sick.

• Type 2 diabetes, as well as nearly every other significant disease, has been related to oxidative stress, making antioxidants a must for a healthy body. Many people are surprised to learn that cinnamon has more antioxidants than some well-known superfoods.

• Without injections, you can obtain a bigger pout by simply sprinkling cinnamon on your lips. To keep your lips soft and hydrated throughout the day, mix a small amount of cinnamon with Vaseline or other oil (vitamin E, coconut, olive, etc.).

• With aging, the proteins that keep our skin supple and elastic become fewer in our bodies' tissues. Many products say they can increase protein production, but cinnamon extract seems to do it without any extra chemicals.

• Some experts think cinnamon may promote hair growth, increasing follicular blood flow to enhance hair follicle growth.

Possible Side Effects

• The short-term health benefits of eating small amounts of cinnamon as a spice or supplement are considered safe for the vast majority of the population. Cinnamon contains coumarin. Many people take the blood thinner warfarin made from this component. Coumarin can cause liver damage and interfere with blood coagulation if consumed excessively. Consult your doctor before adding cinnamon to your diet if you have any medical conditions.

IMMUNE-
BOOSTING HERB

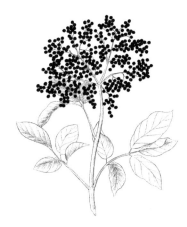

Elderberry (*Sambucus nigra*)

Overview

Supporters of elderberry argue that the fruit is one of nature's most versatile cures. You can find elder trees and plants worldwide in a range of habitats. The elderberry was referred to as a "medicine chest" by Hippocrates, the "Father of Medicine," circa 400 BC. The elderberry is recognized as one of the most healing plants in traditional medicine.

Health advantages

•Elderberry is a low-calorie, high-antioxidant superfood. You can get 106 calories, 26.7 grams of carbs, and barely any fat or protein in one cup of berries. An abundance of antioxidants, such as phenolic acids, found in elderberries can help the body recover from the effects of oxidative stress.

•Black elderberry extracts and flower infusions help reduce influenza symptoms and duration. Elderberry-based cold remedies come in some dosage forms, including pills, tablets, and chewable, in addition to liquids.

•Elderberries are a great source of antioxidants. They assist in the elimination of potentially harmful reactive substances from the body.

•Elderberry consumption may improve some indices of respiratory and heart health. This type of flavonoid, anthocyanins, has been associated with a lower risk of heart disease in people who consume elderberries. It has been found that elderberries can raise insulin levels and reduce blood sugar levels.

•Elderberry inhibits the growth of bacteria like Helicobacter pylori, which may help alleviate sinusitis and bronchitis symptoms. Elderberry polyphenols have been shown to increase the generation of white blood cells. Elderberry extract has been found to have a sun-blocking effect in skin lotions.

Dosing

•Adults are most likely to take daily doses of up to 1200 mg of elderberry fruit extract for two weeks. There are various elderberry products on the market, including syrups and mouthwashes. Medical professionals can help you choose the best product and dose for your specific condition. Elderberries that are not yet ripe should be avoided. They're potentially harmful to your health because of the substances they contain.

Possible Side Effects

●It is generally accepted that little dosages of it are safe. But berries and blossoms that aren't correctly ripe or cooked might cause vomiting, diarrhea, and nausea. Other poisonings might occur when the dosage is increased. Pregnancy and breastfeeding are not recommended times to take this medication. Those with weakened immune systems may be more susceptible to adverse reactions from elderberries.

●If you develop a rash or have difficulty breathing after consuming these substances, you may be allergic to them.

●If you're taking other prescriptions that cause you to pee, you may want to avoid this supplement.

●You should talk to your doctor before eating elderberries.

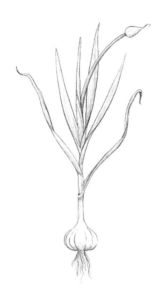

Garlic (Allium sativum)

Overview

Egyptians widely used garlic during the construction of the Giza pyramids about 5,000 years ago. Garlic was recommended by the ancient Greek physician Hippocrates as a treatment for a wide variety of diseases. First, it was through the Indus Valley (the ancient civilizations of Pakistan and western India) where garlic was first cultivated; then, garlic made its way to China from Egypt. Finally, the French, Spanish, and Portuguese carried garlic to the New World, where it quickly became a staple food. Garlic has been used to treat various ailments, including hypertension, diarrhea, gas, and colic. Additionally, it has been used to treat inflammation, diabetes, and tuberculosis (TB) (tuberculosis).

Health advantages

●Eating raw garlic on an empty stomach can alleviate coughs. Rubbing a few cloves of garlic on the back of a child's neck can stop them from coughing.

●Garlic's allicin slows the oxidation of LDL (bad cholesterol). Those with hypertension can benefit from garlic's ability to reduce blood pressure.

●The anti-inflammatory and antioxidant properties of garlic help the brain function better. You can fight Alzheimer's disease with it.

●It assists with digestion when eaten raw. You can remove intestinal worms with the use of garlic tea. In addition to killing unwanted microbes, it preserves good microorganisms.

●The antioxidant-fighting properties of garlic are well-known.

●In addition to clearing acne and reducing scarring, garlic is a potent antioxidant.

●You can use garlic juice to treat rashes, cold sores, and blisters. It also blocks UV radiation, which helps to halt the aging process.

●Antioxidants in garlic also protect against bacterial and fungal diseases. Garlic helps prevent peptic ulcers by removing bacteria from the intestines.

●Garlic inhibits the growth of adipocytes, the cells that store fat. Another advantage is fat burning, which lowers cholesterol levels in the blood through thermogenesis (heating up).

●You may inhibit the growth of E. coli by using garlic juice (UTI). It helps to maintain the health of the kidneys.

●You can reduce bacterial infections by applying garlic to the skin. Garlic in its raw form is used in the majority of home cures.

●You may improve workout endurance by consuming raw garlic fermented in water and alcohol.

●Garlic has been found to help the body recover from being tired after a workout.

●Lead toxicity can be treated most effectively organically with garlic. Most people recommend d-Penicillamine to lower lead levels in the blood, but garlic works better.

●Inconsistent cytokine production during menopause can lead to an estrogen shortage. Garlic use after menopause may help alleviate estrogen insufficiency.

●When it comes to osteoarthritis, garlic consumption can help keep it at bay or even slow its progression. With diallyl disulfide (DDS), which is found in garlic, you can maintain your bone density and avoid bone diseases like osteoarthritis.

●You can reduce platelet stickiness by using garlic. Garlic has been shown to reduce the risk of blood clots and heart attacks.

Possible Side Effects

●You can safely take garlic orally for the vast majority of people. There may be side effects such as bad breath, heartburn, gas, and diarrhea. Taking raw garlic can aggravate these undesirable effects. People who have an allergy to garlic should know they may be at risk of bleeding.

●When applied to the skin, garlic products may be safe. Garlic can cause damage that resembles a burn if applied directly to the skin. Using raw garlic on the skin could be dangerous.

●Garlic can upset some people's stomachs and cause flatulence or diarrhea when taken in large doses.

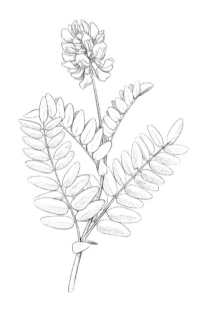

Astragalus (Astralagus)

Overview

This herb is a natural stress reliever. In terms of adaptogens, Astragalus is a great one. It can protect the body from a variety of stresses. In addition to its anti-inflammatory and antioxidant properties, it contains antioxidants that protect cells from oxidation. Astragalus has few side effects when used in low to moderate doses, but it can interact with other plants and prescription medications. Heart disease patients have proven to benefit from its ability to lower cholesterol and improve cardiac function.

Health advantages

●The high antioxidant content of Astragalus makes it a heart-healthy herb. Also, it may help lower cholesterol levels.

●Astragalus root extract is commonly used to treat seasonal allergies. If you have asthma or allergies, the herb astragalus may help relieve your symptoms.

●When it comes to alleviating stress, Astragalus is an excellent choice. You can find antidepressant properties in this ancient herb.

●Using the root of Astragalus can help alleviate insomnia and disrupted sleep patterns. This herb positively impacts the body's overall health, hormonal balance, and metabolism.

●Astragalus' anti-aging properties have made it so important and popular. Facial wrinkles are reduced, tissue growth is accelerated, and signs of chronic illness are averted thanks to this treatment. You may reduce wrinkles and age spots with the use of this root.

●Astragalus has been used for thousands of years to improve the immune system. As a result, the immune system is strengthened, and the body is protected from major harm. Naturally anti-microbial, it can also increase one's resilience to viruses.

Dosage

•There are several variables to consider before prescribing a dosage to a patient. In consultation with your physician, decide on the safest and most effective dosage for you. In higher doses, You can suppress the immune system. Use a standardized astragalus supplement for the greatest results. When taking Astragalus, dosages will vary depending on whether it is utilized as an adaptogen or for other purposes. Patients should talk to a doctor with experience in this area to find the best way to take medicine.

Possible Side Effects

•Astragalus is frequently combined with other herbal products to maximize its benefits. Astragalus appears to have few side effects. In large doses, Astralagus may weaken the immune system. Anyone using an immune-suppressing drug should avoid Astragalus.

•Pregnant or lactating women should not take astragalus root. Those with immune system problems, such as rheumatoid arthritis or lupus, should not use astragalus root.

•Like any herbal supplement, you should always check with your doctor before taking astragalus root pills.

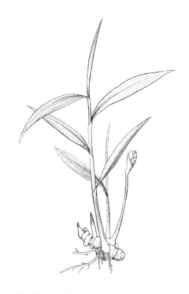

Ginger (Zingiber officinale)

Overview

Ginger is a natural anti-inflammatory. As well as easing nausea and pain, ginger has been shown to treat respiratory problems and reduce flatulence. Ginger also boosts the absorption of calcium, the immune system, and the desire to eat. You can also alleviate weight loss and menstrual cramps with this spicy root. Raw, dehydrated, crushed, oil, and juice are just a few variations. Curries, sauces, and soups in Asian cuisine all feature ginger as a key flavoring agent. Ginger can be found in various foods and beverages, including biscuits, beer, and wine. Since it is now on the FDA's list of generally safe foods, ginger is often added to cough syrups to make them less bitter.

Health advantages

●You can ease pregnancy-induced nausea and vomiting with ginger. Cancer patients may potentially benefit from this treatment for postoperative nausea. It's an anti-seasickness remedy.

●As a home remedy for cardiovascular disease, ginger is an excellent choice. Anti-clotting superfoods include ginger, onion, and garlic. A stroke or a heart attack is less likely if you use these herbs or supplements.

●Ginger relieves post-workout muscle aches and pains. Slowing the growth of muscle soreness might not make the pain go away right away, but it will help.

●Ginger aids digestion and keeps the gastrointestinal tract in good shape. Stomach pains have long been alleviated with the use of this ancient spice. It has a carminative part that helps settle the stomach and get rid of gas.

●Gingerols, the anti-inflammatory compounds found in ginger, are also found in turmeric. Osteoporosis pain is reduced with regular consumption.

●When it comes to your health, ginger is a powerful immune system booster and lymphatic system cleanser. As a result, it flushes out toxins and maintains the body's heat. In addition to boosting your immune system, ginger is also good for your lungs.

●Gingerol, a compound present in ginger, is an effective antifungal and antibacterial agent. S. pyogenes and S. aureus are two bacteria that ginger can combat. Many microbes' growth is inhibited by ginger.

●Ginger has been shown to reduce menstrual cramps. This works equally well as ibuprofen and mefenamic acid. Take one gram of ginger once a day during the first three days of your period. You will reduce menstrual pain by this.

●Improve insulin sensitivity and prevent diabetes with the help of gingerols. By using this supplement, you can avoid diabetes and its complications.

●Ginger: Ginger aids digestion and keeps the stomach healthy. Medications for ulcers do not compare favorably with the effectiveness of this spice.

Dosing

●There are numerous methods to reap the health benefits of ginger. Use freshly minced ginger in your cooking to reap the benefits of ginger while enhancing the flavor of your food. Use ginger in everything from stir-fries to soups to curries; you can even add it to desserts or drinks. Fresh ginger is sometimes included in pre-made tea bags, although these may not be as beneficial to your health as fresh ginger.

Possible Side Effects

•The following is a list of the most frequently reported side effects:

○Diarrhea

○Heartburn

○A distressed stomach, hives

○Swelling

○Breathing difficulties

○It may aggravate acid reflux in certain people.

•This can induce an increase in bile production, leading to the formation of gallstones, which can impede bile flow. Therefore, ginger should be used with caution by patients with gallstone disease since it may increase bile flow.

•Because it can interfere with blood clot formation, you should not take it with blood-thinning medicines like aspirin.

•Even though it is usually safe, women who have had miscarriages in the past should talk to a doctor before making any changes to their diet while pregnant.

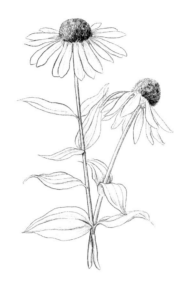

Echinacea (Echinacea purpurea)

Overview

Purple coneflower, another name for echinacea, is a commonly used herbal remedy. Since time immemorial, Native Americans have used it to treat various illnesses. It's well known for its common cold and flu herbal cures. In addition, you can use it to treat inflammation, discomfort, and headaches, among other things.

Health advantages

•You can protect your body's cells from oxidative stress, which is linked to various chronic illnesses, including heart disease, diabetes, and more. Echinacea plants are rich in antioxidant phytochemicals. Some examples include cichoric acid, flavonoids, and rosmarinus acid.

•Echinacea's most well-known usage is as an immune system booster. When used with antiviral treatment, echinacea may cut the number of colds by half.

•Echinacea purpurea extract has been shown to block carbohydrate-digesting enzymes. Eat this, and your blood sugar levels will go down. Additionally, extracts have been shown to improve insulin sensitivity. This is because it decreases insulin resistance by eliminating extra fat from the bloodstream, a risk factor.

•Anxiety affects nearly one in every five adults in the United States. Active compounds in echinacea plants offer anti-anxiety qualities. Some examples are rosmarinic acid, alkoxides, and caffeic acid.

•There's a problem if the inflammation persists for longer than it should. This can lead to long-term health problems such as chronic disease. Many studies have shown that Echinacea can reduce inflammation.

•Many studies have shown that echinacea extracts can slow the growth of cancer cells and even kill cancer cells.

●Cancer cells were killed in a test-tube experiment using echinacea purpurea and chicoric acid.

Dosage

●For the time being, echinacea does not have a standard dosage.

Possible Side Effects

●Short-term use of echinacea supplements appears to be both safe and effective. Some consumers have complained of skin reactions like rashes and hives. Allergy sufferers are more likely to have negative reactions to the plant. If you are taking medicine to weaken your immune system, you should not take echinacea or at least talk to your doctor about it.

●Echinacea has been proven to be safe when taken orally for a short time. People with autoimmune diseases should avoid echinacea.

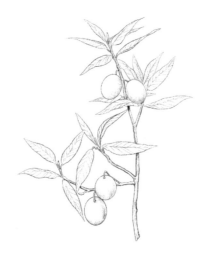

Olive Leaf (Olea europaea)

Overview

Health researchers have discovered that the olive leaf offers many health benefits. Olive leaf extract is a concentrated concentration of the nutrients present in the leaves of the olive tree. Antioxidants in this product will aid your body's natural defenses.

Health advantages

•Olive leaf extract's active ingredient, oleuropein, has been shown in studies to protect against Alzheimer's. Olive leaf extract's ability to fight free radicals may also help with other neurological diseases, like Parkinson's.

●Atherosclerosis, the deadliest form of heart disease, can be prevented by olive leaf extract, according to research. Coronary heart disease is linked to high levels of "bad" LDL cholesterol and total cholesterol.

●Using olive leaf extract as a blood pressure-lowering supplement has been proven to work. In a research investigation, olive leaf extract was found to lower blood pressure. One way to lower one's chance of having a heart attack is to lower one's blood pressure.

●According to a review of studies, olive leaf extract can increase insulin production in cells. One study discovered that patients who took olive leaf extract pills had lower blood sugar and fasting plasma insulin levels. Post-meal insulin levels, on the other hand, were largely unchanged.

●In addition to its heart-healthy characteristics, olive leaf extract has been shown to prevent type 2 diabetes. A high-fat diet was studied to see if olive leaf extract could help prevent obesity. Olive leaf extract may help people lose weight by changing genes associated with weight gain. It can also help you consume fewer calories.

●One study demonstrated that olive leaf extracts slowed the growth of cancerous cells in the laboratory. The extract has been connected to antioxidant effects by experts.

Dosage

●Olive leaf extract supplements are now available in powder form in addition to tablets, soft gels, and tinctures. Between 500 and 1,000 milligrams (mg) of vitamin D a day is sufficient for most people.

●The recommended dosage ranges from 250 to 500 mg per day. You can achieve the optimum outcomes by taking it twice to four times a day with food. Make sure to read the label before using any vitamin. If you choose, you can talk to your doctor about the dosage.

Possible Side Effects

●Some people may have unfavorable side effects from eating olive leaves in tiny doses for a short period. When OLE (olive leaf extract) is used for detoxification, it can cause moderate symptoms, including headaches. If you are on blood pressure medication or have low blood pressure, OLE should be avoided because it can further lower your blood pressure.

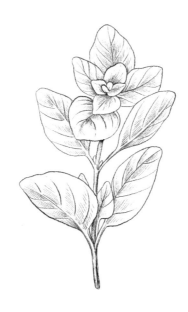

Oregano (Origanum vulgare)

Overview

Lamiaceae, or mint, is the botanical family from which oregano is descended. It has been used as a flavoring and therapeutic element for thousands of years. In the Mediterranean diet, it's a must-have item. The Greeks and Romans viewed oregano as a symbol of joy and happiness. The name was originated because the Greek word "or" means "mountain" and "ganos" means "joy." It's possible to get oregano in a variety of ways. Oregano can be taken as a supplement or in the form of an oil. In addition to terpinene and thymol, caryophyllene and carvacrol are responsible for the herb's flavor and scent. There are various health benefits to oregano oil as well. Incorporated into a person's diet, oregano boosts their antioxidant intake.

Health advantages

•A high concentration of antioxidants in oregano can help minimize the oxidative damage caused by free radicals. Consuming oregano and other high-antioxidant foods, such as fruits and vegetables, may benefit your health.

•Components of oregano have antibacterial properties. In tests in test tubes, researchers found the antibacterial properties of oregano to be effective against 23 different species of bacteria. They found that thyme essential oil killed bacteria the best, but oregano was a close second.

•Scientists have discovered that oregano ingestion may aid in protecting cells from DNA damage. Oregano and its components may be able to fight cancer cells. Oregano extract was shown to stop colon cancer cells from making tumors and also help get rid of tumors that were already there.

•Some research suggests that oregano and its constituents may offer some protection against viruses. Oregano's antiviral properties extend beyond carvacrol and thymol. A single hour of carvacrol therapy immobilized the Norovirus, a virus that causes abdominal pain, diarrhea, and nausea.

●Antioxidants in oregano can also protect against free radical damage. Carvacrol, an anti-inflammatory molecule, has been found in significant concentrations in this plant.

●For the first time, two oregano oil constituents have been shown to have anti-inflammatory properties. Experiments in the lab have shown that oregano extract can help reduce inflammation, which may be a factor in:

○Allergic asthma

○Rheumatoid arthritis

○Autoimmune arthritis

● Type 2 diabetes may benefit from the chemical elements of oregano. A review suggests that using origanum extract may help reduce insulin resistance and modulate gene expression that impacts fat and carbohydrate metabolism.

Possible Side Effects

For the most part, oregano is harmless in all its forms for most people. However, individuals should:

●Supplements should not be taken by anyone currently taking medication or with a medical condition.

•For the two weeks leading up to surgery, avoid oregano foods, as it can increase the risk of bleeding.

•Essential oils should be diluted in a steam bath using water or a carrier oil such as olive oil. If the oregano oil content exceeds 1%, the skin may get inflamed.

•You should never use essential oils on your skin or ingest them. To avoid poisoning, each product must be used exactly as directed.

•It is possible that oregano may interfere with the absorption of copper, iron, and zinc. It's possible that lowering blood sugar levels will also help.

•People who are allergic to plants in the Lamiaceae family should be warned that oregano may cause an allergic reaction.

ADAPTOGENIC HERBS

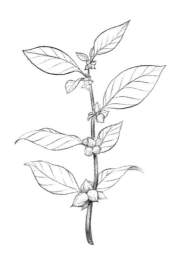

Ashwagandha (Withania somnifera)

Overview

Ashwagandha is native to Asia and Africa. It has velvety leaves and bell-shaped blooms. Ashwagandha's anti-inflammatory and immunostimulatory activities have been linked to several of the plant's constituents. Ashwagandha is utilized as an adaptogen for a variety of stress-related illnesses. Sleeplessness, aging, and anxiety are among the conditions addressed by this herb.

Health advantages

Researchers have found that Ashwagandha can help treat a wide range of illnesses, such as:

●Anxiety and Stress: Ashwagandha is well-known for its ability to support healthy cortisol levels and reduce the body's stress response.

●Ashwagandha can help inhibit the transmission of pain signals to the brain and reduce pain symptoms. Additionally, there may be anti-inflammatory effects.

●Improved hypertension, reduced triglycerides, and alleviated chest tightness are only some of the benefits of Ashwagandha's use in improving cardiovascular health. This can help prevent heart disease.

• Ashwagandha has been studied for its capacity to reduce or prevent cognitive decline for illnesses like Alzheimer's, Huntington's, and Parkinson's disease.

• Studies show that Ashwagandha may be able to slow the growth of cancer cells.

Dosing

The dosage and technique of Ashwagandha's use vary depending on the condition being treated. Capsules of Ashwagandha typically contain between 250 and 1,500 mg of the plant. High doses can produce undesirable side effects in some patients. Before taking any herbal supplement, including ashwagandha, talk to your doctor to ensure it's safe and effective.

Possible Side Effects

Small to moderate quantities of Ashwagandha are generally safe. However, when eaten in excessive amounts, it can produce nausea, vomiting, and diarrhea in the stomach. Ashwagandha should be avoided by expectant mothers and those attempting to conceive because it can induce fetal distress or even miscarriage. Auto-immune disease sufferers should also exercise caution when taking ashwagandha, as it can boost immune system activity and, as a result, the severity of their symptoms. You should not take ashwagandha with any of the following medications:

- Immunosuppressants

- Sedative medications (Benzodiazepines)

- Sedative medications (CNS depressants)

- Thyroid hormone

- Medications for diabetes (Anti-diabetic drugs)

- Medications for high blood pressure (Antihypertensive drugs)

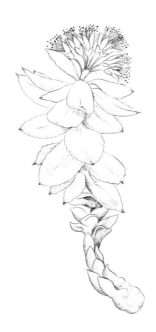

Rhodiola (Rhodiola rosea)

Overview

Flowers of the Rhodiola genus are native to Europe and Asia and thrive in the cold, mountainous regions. This plant's roots function as an adaptogen when eaten internally. As a result, Rhodiola is known as "arctic root" or "golden root" by herbalists around the world. Rosavin and salidroside are the two most powerful active ingredients.

Health Advantages

•Many people know Rhodiola as an adaptogen, a natural substance that boosts the body's ability to deal with stress. Burnout can happen when someone is under a lot of stress for a long time. Rhodiola can help with this.

•Anxiety and Depression: An imbalance of neurotransmitters in the brain causes depression and anxiety. Rhodiola aids in the re-establishment of neurotransmitter balance. A study comparing the effects of Rhodiola to those of sertraline (a common antidepressant) found that while the herb did not reduce symptoms as much as sertraline, it was milder and had fewer side effects.

•Rhodiola may help athletes perform better by lowering fatigue and enhancing antioxidant activity, but the evidence is mixed when it comes to this.

•Some of the symptoms of diabetes, like tiredness and thirst, can be relieved by taking Rhodiola.

- Salidroside, the main part of Rhodiola, is thought to stop cancer cells from growing.

Dosing

Rhodiola should only be taken on an empty stomach and not before bedtime because of its somewhat stimulating qualities. Most of the Rhodiola extract in pills or capsules containing between 100 and 200 mg is made up of Rosavins and salidroside. It's also possible to buy tinctures. A single dose of 400–600 mg of Rhodiola per day, either as a single dose or divided into two doses, may help relieve stress, fatigue, and depression. Several studies have shown that even doses of as little as 200 to 300 mg daily can improve athletic performance. Unfortunately, Rhodiola Rosea extract capsules and tablets are hard to come by. On the other hand, many people prefer taking their medication in pill form because it is easier to control the dosage. It is also available as a herbal tea.

Possible Side Effects

For a period of six to twelve weeks, Rhodiola may be considered safe. However, avoid taking Rhodiola if you experience any of these side effects. Long-term safety research on Rhodiola is lacking. Pregnant or breastfeeding women should not use this product.

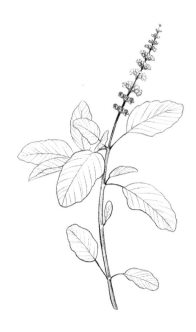

Tulsi, or Holy Basil (Ocimum tenuiflorum)

Overview

Tulsi (Ocimum tenuiflorum), also known as the "Queen of Herbs," is a plant native to Southeast Asia. It has been used in Indian medicine to treat everything from eye disorders to ringworms. In addition, holy basil is said to have therapeutic properties for physical, mental, and spiritual well-being.

Employing different parts of the plant to treat different diseases is possible.

Health advantages

•In addition to vitamin C and zinc, Tulsi is an excellent source of these nutrients. As a result, immunity is boosted, and infections are prevented. It has antiviral, antibacterial, and antibiotic properties that aid in the fight against infection.

•The antibacterial and antiviral properties of tulsi aid in treating illness and reducing the body's temperature. Tulsi includes the anti-inflammatory terpene eugenol, which is abundant in the plant.

•There are antiviral and antibacterial properties in tulsi's camphene, cineole, and eugenol. You can treat asthma, bronchitis, flu, cough, and colds with honey and ginger.

•The ocimum sides A and B of Tulsi are known to lower stress and blood pressure. These molecules alleviate stress and regulate the brain's serotonin and dopamine levels. Because of its anti-inflammatory qualities, it can aid in the reduction of blood pressure.

•To combat cancer, the anti-cancer properties of Tulsi are evident. In other words, they help us avoid skin, liver, mouth, and lung cancer.

•Taking Tulsi, which has antioxidant properties and lowers blood pressure, can help prevent and treat cardiovascular disease.

•It has been shown that Tulsi leaf extract can lower blood glucose levels in type 2 diabetics.

•Gout and kidney stones are helped with tulsi. It is a diuretic and a purifying agent. Kidney stones are caused by an excess of uric acid in the blood. Gout patients can benefit from lowering their uric acid levels.

•Dyspepsia and appetite loss can be treated using the leaves of Tulsi. It is possible to use them to reduce gas and bloating.

•Tulsi aids in the removal of acne and pimples from the skin. The antioxidants in it help the body age gracefully. Tulsi strengthens the teeth.

•When eaten daily, Tulsi also helps to purify the blood.

•Because of its teeth-and gum-strengthening properties, tulsi is an excellent ingredient in herbal toothpaste. You can also use it to treat oral ulcers, so it's a one-stop-shop for all things dental.

•There are numerous health benefits of taking tulsi, both in terms of physical and mental health. It alleviates stress and exhaustion.

Possible Side Effects

•Drink Tulsi tea made from fresh leaves gathered from the plant.

●You can brew fresh tulsi leaves, dried tulsi leaves, or tulsi powder with 1 cup of boiling water for the best tulsi tea. Let the water settle for about 15 minutes in a saucepan or mug before drinking it. After that, strain the tea, sweeten with honey if preferred, and enjoy.

●You can also consume Tulsi pills and powders.

Some Things You Need to Know About Tulsi:

●Women attempting to get pregnant should avoid Tulsi since it may interfere with their ability to get pregnant.

●If drinking tulsi tea makes you sick or gives you diarrhea, start with a small amount and slowly increase it.

●It is important for people with diabetes to be aware of the possible harmful effects of Tulsi.

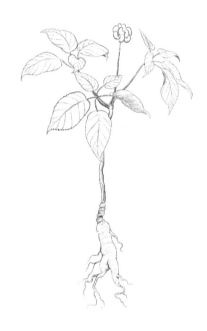

Ginseng (Panax ginseng)

Overview

Ginseng has long been employed in traditional Chinese medicine. Fresh, white, and red varieties of this slow-growing plant are available. Its roots are fleshy, and it develops slowly. It is customary to harvest white ginseng between the ages of 4 and 6, whereas red ginseng is often harvested at the end of the 6 years. Ginsengs from the United States and Asia are the most readily available. American ginseng is different from Asian ginseng in terms of active chemicals and physiological effects. Ginsengs from the United States and Asia have different effects on the body. In ginseng, you'll find ginsenosides and gintonin. Together, these substances can help you stay healthy.

Health advantages

●Ginseng's antioxidant properties can help relieve inflammation. Inflammatory ginseng polysaccharides and ginsenoside components have been shown in various laboratory experiments to reduce inflammation and boost cellular antioxidant capability.

●Taking ginseng could improve your memory, behavior, and temperament. Compound K and ginsenosides, which are contained in ginseng, have been shown to protect against free radical damage to the brain. Other studies have shown an improvement in the brain activity and behavior of Alzheimer's disease patients.

●Ginseng can help erectile dysfunction in men with ginseng. According to studies, ginseng may be helpful for men's erectile dysfunction (ED). Several of its constituent compounds may aid in the restoration of normal function and the prevention of oxidative stress in the penis's blood vessels and tissues. Ginseng helps the muscles and blood vessels in the penile area make more nitric oxide.

●The herb ginseng may also help cancer patients' vaccines work better by making their immune systems stronger.

- Ginseng may help lower the risk of getting a few different kinds of cancer by protecting against free radicals, reducing inflammation, and making cells healthier.

- Ginseng has been shown to stop oxidative damage and increase cellular energy synthesis. This may help people feel less tired and be more active.

- Fermented red ginseng extracts are an excellent source of antioxidant protection.

Dosage

No dose for ginseng has been established. However, dosages have been studied in a wide range. Ginseng dosages can range from 0.2 to 9 grams per day for four to twenty-four weeks.

Possible Side Effects

- Ginseng is commonly used and even found in alcoholic beverages, but this does not mean it is entirely safe. Nevertheless, like with any herbal supplement or prescription, undesirable side effects may occur.

- Only a few of the most common side effects have been reported:

- Headaches

- Problems with digestion

●Insomnia

●People with hypertension (high blood pressure) should not take ginseng supplements unless their doctor tells them to. The combination of diabetes medicines and ginseng may result in a reduction in blood sugar. If you have diabetes, do not take this product without visiting your doctor.

●Children and breastfeeding mothers should avoid using Panax ginseng.

Talk to your doctor if you're taking any medication. Blood sugar levels can be affected by ginseng. For diabetics, this is especially true.

●Other antidepressants, such as warfarin, may also interact with this medicine. In addition, ginseng's stimulant qualities may be boosted by adding caffeine to the formula.

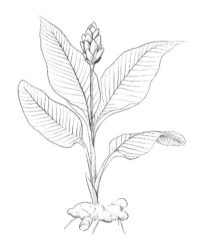

Turmeric (Curcuma)

Overview

Turmeric, a yellow spice, is a potent supplement to a nutritious diet. A dish's color can be attributed to turmeric. Turmeric is an excellent substance for both your physical and mental health. Curcumin, the principal active component, is responsible for these advantages. According to current research, turmeric does indeed contain therapeutic ingredients. Curcuminoids are the building blocks of these substances. In addition, Curcumin, the main ingredient in turmeric, also provides anti-inflammatory effects. In addition to being a potent antioxidant, it also has anti-inflammatory properties.

Health advantages

●The long-term effects of chronic inflammation can be dangerous. Curcumin appears to be able to lower inflammation by preventing the body's production of key inflammatory indicators. Turmeric's antioxidant properties help reduce oxidative stress, which is linked to inflammation.

●Turmeric extract is often used to treat joint pain and arthritis. Joint stiffness, swelling, and decreased mobility are signs of severe arthritis. These symptoms could intensify and lead to permanent damage if ignored. When it comes to illnesses such as rheumatoid arthritis and osteoarthritis, curcumin significantly impacts the inflammatory mediators.

●Turmeric has been shown to ease some of the symptoms of arthritis, which could make it a possible treatment.

●Neuralgia, disc herniation, and other spinal abnormalities are common causes of chronic back pain. There is no cure for these ailments, but studies have shown that turmeric can help reduce inflammation and damage from free radicals.

●Studies have shown that curcumin can stabilize the metabolism and regulate weight in patients with metabolic illnesses. Controlling fat metabolism and suppressing adipose tissue are two of turmeric's primary benefits.

- It has been proven that curcumin can minimize the damage produced by free radicals in inflammatory skin conditions.

- Turmeric also makes collagen and has been shown to speed up the healing of damaged tissues.

- It enhances brain function.

- Lowers Anxiety and Depression

- Asthma and allergy relief

- Aids in Liver Detoxification

- Headaches and Migraines

- Diabetes

- Inflammation of the blood vessels

- Turmeric can help prevent diseases and long-term conditions like Alzheimer's and Parkinson's disease, as well as treat them when they happen.

- Cholesterol regulation

- Candida Infection

- Anxiety-Induced Constipation (IBS)

- Irritable Bowel Syndrome (IBD)

- Myalgic Encephalomyelitis and Chronic Fatigue Disorder

- Thyroid Disorder

Dosing

- Researchers have discovered that taking 1.4 grams of turmeric extract twice daily for three months can reduce cholesterol levels.

- You can treat itching (pruritus) by taking 1500 mg of turmeric in three equal doses over eight weeks.

- People with joint osteoarthritis have reported improvement in their symptoms after taking a turmeric supplement for about four to six weeks.

- You can utilize it in the kitchen for meat and fish dishes.

Possible Side Effects

- It's possible that it'll make you feel sick.

- The digestive-healthy qualities of turmeric may cause some discomfort if taken in high amounts. The production of stomach acid is boosted by turmeric. This may help some people's digestion, but it may not work for everyone.

- In addition, it thins the blood out.

- The cleaning properties of turmeric may result in bleeding. Reduced cholesterol and blood pressure are two other turmeric advantages that may have something to do with the way turmeric interacts with your blood

●Heavy doses of turmeric should be avoided by anyone taking blood thinners such as warfarin.

●Due to turmeric's blood-thinning properties, pregnant women should not take it. Turmeric in small amounts as a spice is safe.

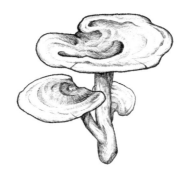

Reishi (Ganoderma lingzhi)

Overview

The Ganoderma fungus (often known as the reishi mushroom) is native to Asia. It has been used in Chinese medicine for generations to treat various ailments. Fresh mushrooms are eaten less often than powdered or extracted mushrooms.

Health advantages

●Because of what it does to white blood cells, this mushroom greatly affects the immune system. White blood cells stop bacteria and cancer from growing.

●This fungus has become a popular food ingredient to combat cancer. The mushroom has been found to be helpful for cancer patients in several trials. Cancer patients saw a rise in their white blood cell activity and improved quality of life.

●Some medical conditions may be helped by reishi mushrooms, which have been shown to help with anxiety and depression and improve overall health.

●In studies, reishi mushrooms increased "good" HDL cholesterol levels while decreasing bad LDL cholesterol levels.

●Chemicals found in the reishi mushroom have been shown in several tests to reduce blood sugar levels.

Dosage

Unlike other foods or supplements, the dosage of reishi mushrooms varies depending on the type. The largest doses are found in the mushroom itself. Doses might vary from 25 to 100 grams depending on the mushroom size. Typically, a powdered mushroom extract is utilized instead. This method uses a ten-fold lower dose than if the mushroom is ingested.

A 50-gram serving of reishi mushrooms equals about 2 tablespoons of the mushroom extract. Starting with 1.5–9 grams of mushroom extract daily is a good place to begin.

On the other hand, some supplements merely use a small portion of the extract. Certain scenarios necessitate lower suggested doses. You must know the mushroom's shape if you want the greatest outcomes.

Possible Side Effects

•If you consume reishi mushrooms for more than three to six months, you may have an allergic reaction that causes dry skin.

•It can also cause:

•Dizziness

•Itchiness

•Rash

•Headaches

•Stomach upset

•Nosebleed

•Bloody stools

People with low blood pressure may be more at risk from ingesting reishi mushrooms than ever before. Reishi mushrooms may also interfere with high blood pressure medications.

EXPECTORANT HERBS

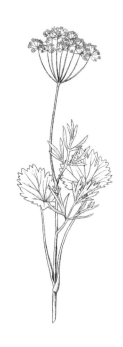

Anise seed (Pimpinella anisum)

Overview

Many people utilize anise (Pimpinella anisum) for medicinal purposes, which has been around for a long time. One of the most potent spices is anise seed. People are familiar with it because of its characteristic licorice flavor. When it comes to cuisine, anise dates back as far as ancient Egypt. To aid in digestion, the Romans ate anise seed cakes. Besides the seeds and oil, anise's roots and leaves can also be used for medical purposes. Anise is widely used in various products, including food and drink, confections, and breath fresheners. Its aroma is also found in other cosmetics, including soaps, lotions, and even sachets. Anise, celery, and parsley all have antiseptic qualities. It is common to use anise as a flavoring agent in desserts and beverages because of its licorice flavor. It is well-known for how well it improves health and works as a natural cure for a wide range of illnesses and problems.

Health advantages

●Vitamins and minerals abound in anise seed. Anise seed contains omega 3 and 6 fatty acids, dietary fiber, sodium, and potassium, which are essential for your body. Calcium, iron, zinc, copper, magnesium, and selenium are all found in anise seed.

•Free radical damage to healthy cells significantly contributes to many types of cancer in our bodies. Consuming anise seeds, which are high in antioxidants, can help prevent this.

•There's a lot of vitamin C and antioxidants in anise seeds, which are helpful for our immune system as a whole. Healthy cells are shielded from oxidative damage by the antioxidant properties of vitamins C and A. Vitamin C also helps make more white blood cells, which is positive for the immune system.

•Our skin benefits from anise seed's high levels of vitamin C and B vitamins, as well as minerals such as phosphorus and zinc.

•We need Vitamin C to protect our skin from oxidative damage, which causes wrinkles, dark spots, and other signs of aging.

•Vitamin A is produced in our bodies from beta-carotene, which is found in anise seeds. The antioxidant capabilities of vitamin A are essential for preventing free radical damage to our eye cells.

•Preventing age-related macular degeneration, as well as night blindness and cataracts, have all been linked to anise seed consumption.

•Eating anise seeds can improve your overall health and minimize your risk of developing diabetes. By keeping sugar from being absorbed into the body as quickly as it should be, fiber-rich anise seeds help to reduce blood sugar levels.

•Anemia is a condition that occurs when the body does not have enough iron. So, consuming anise seed and other iron-rich foods can help boost our iron levels and lower our risk of anemia.

•Calcium, copper, manganese, and phosphorus are all excellent for our bones, and anise seed contains all of them. Those who regularly consume calcium-rich foods like anise seeds have a lower risk of developing bone diseases like osteoporosis.

•Anise seed has anti-inflammatory properties due to its high copper concentration.

•You can reduce inflammation caused by disorders like arthritis when ingesting anise seeds daily.

•A wide variety of diseases have been alleviated by using anise seed tea. Asthma, bronchitis, and catarrh are all prevented.

•Anise seed has a high potassium concentration, dilating blood vessels and arteries, reducing the burden on them. Anise seed and other potassium-rich foods have been demonstrated to help lower blood pressure and prevent disorders like hypertension.

Dosage

•Oil, powder, and extract are all forms of anise that can be purchased in addition to dry seeds.

•In baked goods and candy, as well as soaps and lotions, anise can be used in various ways.

•A few teaspoons of ground anise seed, oil, or extract are usually all that is needed in most recipes.

Possible Side Effects

•The vast majority of people can safely consume anise without experiencing any adverse effects.

•Fennel and celery are in the same family as parsley, so they may cause an allergic reaction in people who are sensitive to plants in this family.

•By mimicking the estrogenic effects of breast cancer and endometriosis, anise may worsen the symptoms of both diseases. If you have a family history of any of these disorders, discuss your concerns with your doctor.

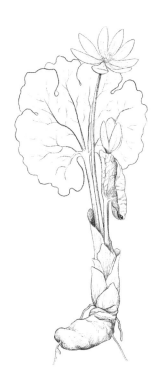

Bloodroot (Sanguinaria canadensis)

Overview

In North America, Bloodroot (Sanguinaria canadensis) is a common wildflower. Bloodroot has been used for centuries as a blood cleanser to cure fevers and slow-healing wounds. Slices of the bloodroot plant's branches and tubers reveal a blood-orange fluid, hence the name "bloodroot." With the plant's nutrient-dense juices, stems, and roots, indigenous people used the plant to dye everything from baskets to garments to battle paint. In addition, bloodroot plant components have been demonstrated to aid with a wide range of health conditions, including colds, sinus infections, high blood pressure, and various skin ailments, among others.

Health advantages

•You can find an ingredient in Bloodroot known as sanguinarine in the plant. Prostate cancer cells have been found to reduce in size after taking this supplement.

•It's possible that Bloodroot can slow the progression of skin cancer cells. This black salve is applied topically to the skin to help prevent the development of cancerous growths.

•Gingivitis and other gum infections benefit significantly from the antibacterial properties of Bloodroot, a common ingredient in toothpaste. In addition, plaque on teeth is less likely to accumulate, and oral health is better.

•Flu, colds, lung infections, and a variety of sinus problems have been treated with Bloodroot for years. In addition, you can clear phlegm and mucus out with the help of this expectorant.

●In part because of its chemical components, Bloodroot has been linked to various cardiovascular conditions. This approach can slow or prevent atherosclerosis.

●Antioxidants and anti-inflammatory components in Bloodroot are utilized in skin lotions and herbal medicines to treat eczema and skin lesions such as psoriasis, acne, and warts.

●The anti-inflammatory properties of Bloodroot make it a good choice for migraines and headaches.

●This is an excellent treatment for people with arthritis. Pain and inflammation in the joints can be relieved with bloodroot paste, which also promotes circulation, encourages the production of new cells, and maintains a healthy metabolic rate in the body.

Dosage

Research on Bloodroot is still in its infancy, so it's hard to give precise dosage recommendations. Depending on the harvest, season, and plant, the efficiency of its plant components might vary nearly tenfold. However, at doses below five mcg, sanguinarine, an alkaloid in Bloodroot, is safe and valuable.

Possible Side Effects

Bloodroot is generally safe as a short-term dietary supplement, but some people may have gastrointestinal upset. When applied topically, Bloodroot can cause adverse skin reactions such as rashes and edema. Overuse of sanguinarine, the poison bloodroot, can result in severe consequences. Signs of sanguinarine poisoning include:

- Blurred vision

- An abnormally slow heartbeat

- Vomiting

- Nausea

- Fainting

- Dizziness

- Eyeballs dilated

- Diarrhea

Anyone experiencing the following signs and symptoms should visit a doctor immediately.

- Pregnant women and children under six should not consume Bloodroot. In addition, people with low blood pressure or cardiac rhythm disorders should not take this drug.

●Bloodroot may affect anti-arrhythmic, blood-thinning, and anti-hypertensive medications.

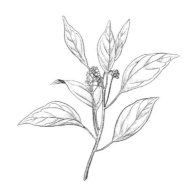

Camphor (Cinnamomum camphora)

Overview

Wood from camphor trees can be distilled using steam distillation. Camphor is a wax-like substance with a pungent odor that is commonly used to treat skin conditions.

Cosmetics and personal care products such as lotions, creams, toothpaste, and deodorants contain it because it is an organic compound. Pain, itching, and irritation can all be relieved by rubbing a little on the skin.

Additionally, camphor can help alleviate chest congestion and inflammatory conditions. You can quickly inhale the foul odor and taste of this chemical. Turpentine oil is a common ingredient in the manufacturing of camphor. The use of oral camphor is harmful. When applied to exposed wounds, camphor can reach deadly levels quickly. Small amounts of camphor applied to the affected area can provide relief from pain and itching. In addition, it helps relieve nasal congestion by producing a cooling sensation in your nose.

Health advantages

•The FDA permits the topical application of 3–11% camphor concentrations as a pain reliever. Ointments for osteoarthritis may contain it.

•You can alleviate skin irritation or itching by applying 3–11% camphor to the affected area. Hemorrhoids, bug bites, and cold sores can all be cured with this substance.

•Camphor concentrations greater than 11% are not permitted in FDA-approved chest massages. Using camphor oil to relieve chest congestion is a common practice in aromatherapy.

●Applying camphor to the scalp relieves itching caused by dandruff. This substance can be found in various over-the-counter dandruff shampoos and treatments.

●The use of menthol, camphor, and eucalyptus oil may help reduce the size of mosquito bites and rashes when applied topically. If you add virgin coconut oil to the mix, it will be less irritating to the skin.

●Many people use mothballs made of camphor to keep moth larvae out of clothing and storage facilities.

Possible Side Effects

●Most adults can safely use a cream, balm, or lotion containing a diluted form of camphor. The use of camphor may result in minor adverse effects, such as skin irritation and redness. Don't massage in the cream or lotion that contains camphor. The skin can become irritated if the concentration of camphor is greater than 11 percent. The eyes and mouth should not be exposed to camphor compounds at all. You should not use camphor-containing products on skin that has been damaged or injured. Camphor can easily be absorbed by the skin, which could be dangerous.

●You should avoid the consumption of all forms of camphor at all costs. It's harmful and has the potential to have significant consequences, such as:

○Mouth stinging

○Vomiting and feeling sick

○Seizures

○Confusion

○Disruptions in vision

●Women who are pregnant or nursing should avoid using camphor.

●You should keep products containing camphor away from children at all times. There is a chance that they will cause convulsions. Also, do not apply them to the skin of children. Children are more sensitive to the irritants in camphor than adults.

●If you have a liver issue, avoid using any products that include camphor. It has the potential to make the condition worse.

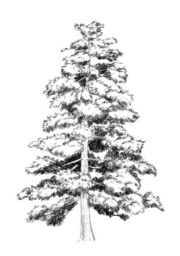

Cedar (Cedrus)

Overview

Native Americans used cedar oil to increase spiritual communication, make people happy, and protect them from evil things. To extract cedarwood oil, you can use steam distillation, cold pressing, or carbon distillation processes. In ancient Egyptian folklore, Egyptians reputedly used this oil for embalming mummies because of its sweet, woody, warm, and comforting scent, which the ancient Egyptians believed was a powerful aid for their passage to the afterlife. You can use cedarwood essential oil if you suffer from many skin issues. It can also be used in aromatherapy and other massage treatments and to treat inflammatory ailments like arthritis and respiratory disorders. For renal problems, it's also a good choice.

Health advantages

●As a sedative and mood enhancer, cedarwood essential oil is ideal for relieving anxiety and its accompanying symptoms, such as restlessness, agitation, and cold hands and feet. People are happier and more optimistic when they are calm and grounded.

●It helps remove impurities and excess oils from the skin while protecting it against germs, preventing infections, irritation, and peeling. Cedar tree essential oil is particularly useful in treating eczema and seborrheic rashes due to its various active components and antibacterial properties. Antioxidants also protect the skin, and wrinkles are delayed by a few years.

●For all your hair woes, cedarwood essential oil is a one-stop shop because of its wealth of bioactive compounds. Hair follicles benefit from enhanced blood flow, protection from several hair infections, and active participation in collagen production because of this oil's antimicrobial characteristics. This substance can aid in treating dandruff, alopecia, and hair thinning in several ways. Regular application of the oil results in improved hair quality, radiance, and thickness. Stress-reducing properties help to prevent hair loss and premature graying of hair.

●Inflammation of the joints and surrounding tissues is caused by arthritis. Cedarwood essential oil's anti-inflammatory and pain-reducing properties make it a great pain reliever. It is also used to treat muscle spasms, aches and pains, headaches, and other inflammatory illnesses since it dilates the blood vessels.

•Several bioactive parts of cedarwood essential oil have been shown to help treat upper respiratory tract illnesses like the common cold and flu. Also, it can alleviate the symptoms of pharyngitis, a sore throat, and other respiratory ailments.

Dosage

•The correct amount of cedar to use depends on various factors, including the user's age and health. Natural products aren't always safe, and it's important to remember that quantities can be critical. Always check with a pharmacist or doctor before using any product and follow the instructions on the label.

Possible Side Effects

•Food additives and pesticides are safe to use if they contain cedarwood oil. Dilution is necessary before applying an essential oil to the skin. Before using the oil, test a small area of your skin to ensure it won't irritate it. Avoid using cedarwood oil if you have an allergy to cedar.

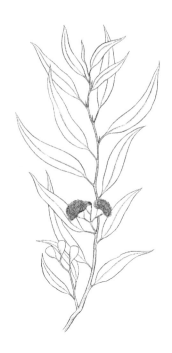

Eucalyptus (Eucalyptus)

Overview

The medicinal properties of eucalyptus are derived from the oil extracted from the tree's oval-shaped leaves, which are used to make the oil. Essential oils can be extracted from leaves, applied to the skin, or breathed in. The essential oil is extracted from the leaves by drying, crushing, and distilling them. Flavonoids and tannins, both plant-based antioxidants, are also found in the leaves. It is employed as a solvent in the industry, as a flavoring agent, as a flavoring ingredient in cosmetics, and as an antiseptic and an antibacterial in eucalyptus oil. A wide range of ailments has been treated with it for thousands of years in Chinese, Indian, Greek, and other European medical systems.

Health advantages

●Research demonstrates that inhaling eucalyptus oil for five minutes helps people with upper respiratory tract infections feel better and improves nasal airflow.

●Those with dyssomnia and a diminished sense of smell can benefit from using this oil for sleep.

●You can apply eucalyptus oil to many different regions of the body. This oil prevents malaria, tick-borne typhus, and Lyme disease.

●According to the available studies, eucalyptus essential oils have been demonstrated to reduce pain by modifying brain activity and blocking pain-inducing chemicals in the nerves. Topical anesthetic creams commonly contain this ingredient. It's a great pain reliever for hurting joints when administered straight to them.

●A clinical investigation indicated that patients inhaling eucalyptus oil after a knee replacement operation experienced reduced discomfort. Aromatherapy can lower blood pressure by inhaling the essential oil's scent.

•The use of eucalyptus oil before undergoing surgery can assist a patient in feeling at rest, tranquil, and calm.

•The research found that gingivitis, an infection of the gums, was reduced by eucalyptus. The plaque was also reduced as a result.

•Eucalyptus oil can help with herpes simplex virus-induced cold sores. In terms of antiviral activity, eucalyptus outperforms over-the-counter drugs like acyclovir.

Possible Side Effects

Even though eucalyptus leaves are safe for people to eat, breathing in the oil could be bad for your health. It is essential to mention that children's bodies are more exposed to the harmful effects of chemicals. There hasn't been enough research on eucalyptus oil to know if it's safe to take while pregnant or nursing. When eucalyptus oil is applied to the skin, it might cause contact dermatitis in certain people. Before applying essential oils to your skin, use a carrier oil such as fractionated coconut or jojoba oil to prevent irritation. Before using a product, perform a skin patch test to ensure you are not allergic to it. Eucalyptus oil may interfere with medications for high cholesterol, acid reflux, or mental disease. Use it only if necessary after checking with your doctor.

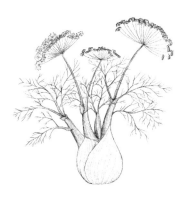

Fennel (Foeniculum vulgare)

Overview

Fennel is a fragrant Mediterranean herb prized for centuries for its flavor and medicinal benefits. Besides being used in cooking, fennel and its seeds have many health benefits, such as anti-inflammatory, antioxidant, and antibacterial properties.

Health advantages

•Fennel seeds contain an antibacterial essential oil. When you eat fennel seeds, your mouth makes more saliva, which helps kill microorganisms.

•Digestive juices move more quickly when fennel seed essential oils are used.

•Fennel seeds have antispasmodic and anti-inflammatory properties, which can help with bloating, nausea, and constipation.

•The potassium in fennel seeds helps maintain a healthy blood pressure level. As a result, blood pressure and heart rate are lowered as well.

•The phytonutrients help feminine hygiene in fennel seeds. Eating these seeds can help with asthma and bronchitis.

•The anethole activates Catalogs, molecules that increase milk production in fennel seeds. Anatole, a hormone made by the thyroid gland, has been shown to make women want to breastfeed.

•Free radical damage to the skin's cells is lessened using fennel extract's antioxidant properties. Potassium, selenium, and zinc are abundant in fennel. These minerals aid in hormone regulation and oxygen balance in the blood.

•If you eat fennel seeds can help get rid of toxins from your body.

•Fennel seeds have been shown to have anti-cancer properties. As potent antioxidants, they protect the body from the harmful effects of oxidative stress. As a result, cancer may be unable to spread.

●When consumed internally, fennel seeds have been demonstrated to improve vision. Fennel seeds are a good source of vitamin A, which is vital for eye health.

●Fiber-rich fennel seeds have been linked to reduced hunger and weight loss. They're diuretic and metabolically active. The high fiber content of fennel seeds makes them an appetite suppressor. This may facilitate weight loss and avoid overeating.

●Fennel seeds have been used for a long time as a digestive aid and antibacterial that can help relieve stomach pain. This seed's digestive action eases bowel movement without causing excessive gas.

Possible Side Effects

●Pregnant women should avoid taking supplements or ingesting the plant's essential oil from fennel. To avoid potential interactions between fennel and other medications, it is recommended that you see your doctor before taking excessive quantities of the herb.

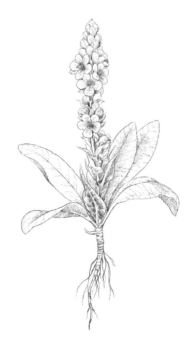

Mullein (Verbascum)

Overview

It has been used in natural therapy to treat mules' ailments for years. Mullein is a popular vegetable. Although most gardeners consider it a weed, herbalists use the flowers and leaves of this plant to treat respiratory and skin conditions. Mullein can also be used to flavor alcoholic beverages, such as beer and whiskey. Pharmaceutical manufacturers rely on the mullein plant for their wares. Oral mullein is used to treat various respiratory ailments, such as asthma and pneumonia. In addition, mullein is used as a flavoring ingredient in the manufacturing of alcohol.

Health advantages

●According to studies, using amantadine and mullein can help prevent influenza A and herpes infections.

●Mullein leaf has been shown to have antibacterial properties against Coli, Staphylococcus aureus, and Klebsiella pneumonia. The dried and natural versions of the leaf or flower are frequently used to make creams and herbal medicines. Numerous naturalists and herbalists utilize mullein to treat respiratory and inflammatory lung conditions.

●In laboratory experiments, mullein has been demonstrated to combat flu-causing viruses.

●Children with earaches can benefit from mullein, garlic, and St. John's Wort ear drops. Lavender and olive oil ear drops can also help.

Possible Side Effects

●Contact dermatitis, a skin reaction that causes itching, redness, and irritation, can be induced by some mullein species. Before applying mullein to your skin, do a patch test to see whether you have any allergic reactions. Research indicates that this product should not be used by women who are or will be pregnant or nursing.

Astringent Herbs

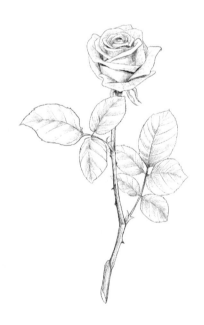

Rose (Rosa)

Overview

Roses have long been revered for their aesthetic and therapeutic properties. Rose tea, a fragrant herbal beverage made from the flowers' petals and buds, is a popular summertime treat. This tea originated in the Middle East and has since become a worldwide sensation. The presence of antioxidants, polyphenols, vitamins A and C, different minerals, myrcene, quercetin, and other compounds in high concentrations is why this tea's numerous health benefits. In addition, Rosebud tea has been used to cure various ailments in traditional Chinese and other complementary medicine systems.

Health advantages

●Anti-inflammatory antioxidants are found in roses. Rose tea has been shown to reduce inflammation, which is linked to weight gain, so it seems logical that it could aid weight loss. For those looking for a caffeine-free alternative to coffee or tea, rose petals can be utilized in the form of a healthy, caffeine-free tea.

●Rose tea has been used for a long time to help with constipation and diarrhea. It does this by making good bacteria grow in the digestive tract.

●Rose tea's ability to flush out toxins and make you urinate less could probably reduce the number of UTIs.

•Stress and anxiety may be alleviated by drinking rose tea.

•Have a horrible period? Cramping around this time of the month might be eased by drinking a cup of warm rose tea. Compared to over-the-counter drugs, rose tea has been shown to have a calming effect on both menstrual cramps' physical and mental symptoms.

•Rose petals and hips are rich sources of antioxidants. Antioxidants protect cells from the destructive effects of free radicals to keep them healthy.

•The antibacterial properties of rose petals can protect you from bacteria. Rose flower extract has also been shown to alleviate inflammation. Rose tea's anti-inflammatory properties may help with several conditions, such as arthritis and other forms of chronic inflammation.

Possible Side Effects

•Excessive drinking of rose tea may cause nausea or diarrhea, according to anecdotal evidence. However, rose extracts are often safe. The FDA has determined that they are safe for human consumption. It's best to check with your doctor before drinking rose tea if you're concerned about your food allergies.

●For most people, one or two cups of relatively strong rose tea should be plenty. Pregnant and lactating women should avoid this tea.

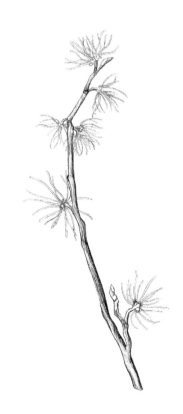

Witch hazel (Hamamelis)

Overview

Known as the witch hazel shrub, Hamamelis virginiana is indigenous to the United States. When treating skin ailments, Native Americans rely heavily on witch hazel. It has been approved by the Food and Drug Administration to be used in over-the-counter drugs. You can make ointments and teas from the bark and leaves. For a long time, witch hazel has been known to relieve inflammation and soothe irritated skin.

Health advantages

•Polyphenols in witch hazel may help fight the aging process. UV [rays] and oxidizing air pollution can hurt the skin. Witch hazel may help because it is an antioxidant.

•The protein-clumping, constricting components of witch hazel cause the proteins in your skin cells to constrict, giving the appearance of smaller pores.

•Tannins found in witch hazel leaves and bark can reduce the appearance of inflamed, red, or blotchy skin.

•The antioxidants and tannins in witch hazel make it an excellent astringent. This aids in the removal of excess oil from the skin.

•The astringent properties of witch hazel help reduce oiliness and redness on the skin. The tannins also provide antibacterial effects in witch hazel.

•You may use witch hazel to level out your skin tone in various ways. Witch hazel has anti-inflammatory and skin-tightening properties.

•After each bowel movement, apply a topical ointment of witch hazel to cure hemorrhoids.

Dosage

•Ointments, gels, and pads containing witch hazel are available. You should avoid products like these if your skin is susceptible. Because of this, product labels may say not to use it more than six times daily. Witch hazel is helpful for some people regularly, while it is only necessary for others on rare occasions. It depends on the individual.

Possible Side Effects

•Skin irritation and allergic reactions can occur if witch hazel is applied directly to the skin, and high amounts may result in nausea and vomiting in the case of ingestion. Only take small doses by mouth; if you notice any bad effects, call your doctor.

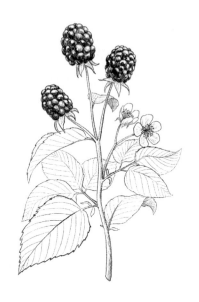

Blackberry Leaf (Rubus fruticosus)

Overview

You can alleviate many ailments by drinking blackberry leaf tea. Anti-inflammatory and antibacterial antioxidants abound in every leaf of this tea. The most excellent part about making blackberry leaf tea is that you may use leaves you've picked from your vines. You just need a few simple ingredients to brew your blackberry leaf tea. The plant's leaves, roots, and fruit are used to make medicine. You can use blackberries to treat various ailments, including diarrhea, fluid retention, diabetes, gout, pain and swelling (inflammation), cancer prevention, and heart disease prevention. It works well as a mouthwash.

Health advantages

•Blackberries are a good source of flavonoid compounds. The antioxidant and anti-inflammatory properties of flavonoids are just two of their many health benefits. Blackberry leaves can be used to treat sore throats, mouth sores, diarrhea, cuts, and hemorrhoids.

•Drinking blackberry leaf tea can kill the H. pylori bacterium.

•Antioxidants found in blackberry leaf tea have been demonstrated to improve general health and well-being.

•Antioxidants found in nature can significantly reduce the risk of developing diseases like cancer. Aside from cancer prevention, antioxidants may also reduce the risk of cardiovascular disease. Antioxidants can be a great addition to a healthy diet.

•This remedy can cure diarrhea, menstrual cramps, and anemia. Leaf decoctions can be used to treat both thrush and bad breath. The leaves of blackberry bushes are a rich source of chlorogenic acid (CGA).

Possible Side Effects

●If you drink too much blackberry leaf tea, you risk experiencing unpleasant side effects like nausea and diarrhea. If you have a medical condition or are taking prescribed medication, it's always better to be safe than sorry. Women who are pregnant or breastfeeding should likewise proceed with caution.

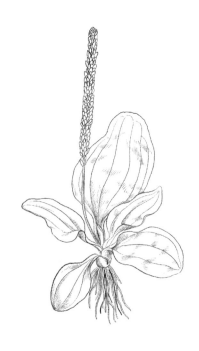

Plantain (Plantago major)

Overview

It is scientifically known as Plantago major, a large-leaved plant that grows across Europe and Asia. It's a drug used to treat various ailments. For centuries, people have relied on the medicinal properties of this plant. The chemicals in plantain weed may help with swelling, digestive problems, and wound healing. Some substances in great plantain may help alleviate pain and swelling, reduce mucus, and clear airways. As far as bacteria and fungus are concerned, it has the potential to kill them. Coughs, mouth sores, obesity, abnormal menstruation cycles, and more can all be treated with large plantains. They seem to like bananas but peeling and eating them is far more complicated.

Health advantages

●Plantain seeds have been found to have anti-inflammatory and cancer-fighting qualities and are used to treat various diseases caused by chronic inflammation. Despite this, plantain weed should not be viewed as a cancer treatment. Human trials are needed to confirm the anti-inflammatory effects of this plant.

●Inflammation, microbial growth, and discomfort can all be reduced using plantain in wound healing. In a study involving

40 participants, aloe vera gel and plantain weed gel were both beneficial in the treatment of foot ulcers.

●Psyllium, a natural laxative, can be found in the seeds of the plantain weed. Plantain leaves can be used to help treat diarrhea and maintain bowel regularity by slowing down the movement of your digestive tract. Plantain extract can be used to treat ulcers.

Possible Side Effects

Eating cooked or raw plantain weed leaves is a safe option for the vast majority of otherwise healthy people. However, plantain supplements have been linked to mild adverse effects like diarrhea and rashes. An allergic reaction that could be fatal is more likely to happen if you take a lot of the medicine.

How to use plantain

●Plantain is available in tincture and tea in pharmacies and health food stores. Aim for three to four servings a day, or roughly five ounces (or 150 mL), to get the most out of infusions and teas. 3–5 grams of powdered medication is a typical daily dosage.

●It's possible to consume both the young and older leaves of plantain weed raw or cooked, depending on the recipe. To use them topically, dry the leaves and infuse them with your preferred oil, such as coconut or sunflower.

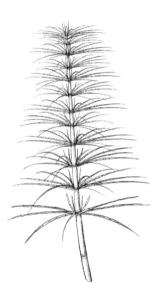

Horsetail (Equisetum)

Overview

Using horsetail as a natural cure dates back to at least Roman times. Skin, hair, and bone health are among the most common uses. "Horse herb" and "bottlebrush" are other names for this plant. Horsetail is anti-inflammatory and antioxidant. Horsetail is used to treat many conditions, such as fluid retention, urinary tract infections, arthritis, and incontinence. In addition, a lot of people believe that horsetail is effective at removing waste and healing wounds.

Health advantages

●Horsetail extract has been demonstrated to increase bone density when taken regularly. This is because the extract has a lot of silica, which helps make collagen and makes it easier for bone and cartilage tissue to absorb and use calcium.

●More urine is excreted from the body when you take diuretics. Herbalists have revered the fern's horsetail for millennia. Dried horsetail extract from a tablet or capsule reduced the number of water people drank.

●If you have nail psoriasis, horsetail extract can cure skin problems in nail lacquer.

●Due to its high content of antioxidants, dry horsetail possesses anti-inflammatory and anti-aging qualities. Hair loss and brilliance are reduced because hair fibers contain more silicon.

Dosage

●Horsetail extract capsules containing 900 mg can have diuretic effects if used for four days.

Possible Side Effects

●Pregnant and lactating women should avoid using horsetail, even though the FDA has not approved it. This plant may cause pharmacological interactions with HIV antiretroviral medicines if used simultaneously. Because it contains nicotine, it is harmful to those who are allergic to it or trying to quit smoking.

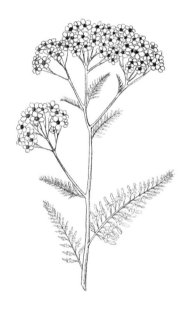

Yarrow (Achillea millefolium)

Overview

Yarrow has been utilized in traditional medicine since the dawn of time. Yarrow has been used as a beverage, skin treatment, and even a flavoring agent in dishes for centuries. Its anti-inflammatory effects alleviate inflammatory conditions. In contrast to the leaves, the flowers of yarrow plants are commonly employed in herbal medicine. Yarrow is frequently used to treat eczema, irritable bowel syndrome (IBS), and skin wounds. People often call yarrow "bloodwort," but this is different from "bloodroot."

Health advantages

•Yarrow has anti-inflammatory chemicals that assist in maintaining the skin's pH and moisture balance. Yarrow is an essential ingredient in many medical lotions because of this. You can use this to reduce bleeding and dull discomfort in powdered form. Studies have shown that yarrow oil works well for treating burns caused by flammable liquids used in warfare.

•As an emmenagogue (a natural cure for menstruation), Yarrow has been used for millennia.

•Yarrow may provide comfort for people who suffer from anxiety and insomnia. It has been demonstrated to provide anti-anxiety effects when supplied to subjects for short and long periods. It also has the same impact as diazepam, an anti-anxiety medication.

•It is thought to contain flavonoids and sesquiterpene lactones that alleviate inflammation.

•Women with mastitis benefit tremendously from Yarrow's use. You can achieve instantaneous pain relief by applying poultices made from the plant's leaves.

●It has been proved that Yarrow has a calming effect on digestion and smooth muscular contractions. The antispasmodic actions of this plant are most likely due to its flavonoid components.

●Yarrow has been associated with reduced blood pressure and enhanced breathing.

Possible Side Effects

●Oral administration of Yarrow can result in drowsiness and increased urination. When used topically, it has the potential to induce skin irritation or dermatitis.

●If you are allergic to ragweed or daisies in the Aster family, you may have a bad reaction to this herb.

●Because the oil has thujone, you should be very careful when using it.

●Coumarin, which has blood-thinning qualities, is also found in this herb. It would be best if you did not take blood-thinning pharmaceuticals with this drug.

●If you are pregnant, you shouldn't use it. If you're pregnant or breastfeeding, talk to your doctor before using yarrow supplements. If you're thinking of using it on your child, talk to your child's doctor first.

In addition, the following drugs may be affected by it:

•Anticoagulants (like warfarin)

•Lithium

•Acid-reducing drugs for the stomach (like omeprazole)

•Medication for hypertension

•Sleep-inducing medications (like anticonvulsants and sleeping pills)

•If you have a history of chronic illness or are taking any drugs, talk to your doctor.

STEP TWO: GET YOUR HERBS

A GUIDE TO GROW HERBS AT HOME

A guide to growing herbs at home

Finding the ideal location for herb gardening

Plant herbs as close as possible to the kitchen. If they're within easy reach, you're considerably more likely to use them. In addition, most herbs require a lot of sunlight to thrive. While rosemary, thyme, basil, and sage are hardy enough to handle full sun, delicate herbs like coriander and parsley should be kept in the shade. Chives and mint will thrive in both settings.

Herb pots, planters, and raised beds

Soggy, chilly soil is the enemy of most herbs that come from dry, hot climates. Garden soil that isn't naturally light and free-draining may be better suited to these plants in raised beds or containers, where you have greater control over the soil mix. A third horticultural grit, or perlite, can be added to raised beds to keep water from rotting the roots for more extended periods. Thyme and rosemary may thrive in pots on a patio or hung from a wall or fence, and they look fantastic. Any container will do, but terracotta is ideal because the clay is porous, preventing the compost from becoming too wet. Many herbs, such as basil (especially Greek), thyme, oregano, chives, curly parsley, and coriander, are naturally compact and can be grown in pots as small as 20cm in diameter. Then, add a third of horticultural grit or perlite, followed by John Innes 2 or 3 soil-based compost.

Herbs to grow

A brilliant place to start is by growing your food. Choose these herbs if you frequently buy parsley, basil, and coriander. Thyme, mint, rosemary, and a gorgeous evergreen potted bay tree—the leaves of which may be used in soups and stews—are all good additions. Then, if you're feeling adventurous, try some less common ingredients, such as chervil, sweet cicely, winter savory, tarragon, and dill. Next, try purple basil, tricolor sage, or tall, feathery fennel for striking aesthetics. What about chocolate mint or lime mint? They're both wonderful alternatives to Bowles's mint. Lemon or orange thyme is much more aromatic than common thyme. Aromatic sages, like blackcurrant or pineapple, have exquisite flavors and produce excellent syrups for cocktails. Add some lemon verbena leaves to boiling water for a refreshing digestif or grow shiso to make purple martins in your backyard.

How to harvest

It's essential to keep snipping your herbs regularly to keep them healthy. You can damage the old brown wood itself, so you should trim only a few leaves or a young bud away from the top of the plant to encourage recovery. There are only a few exceptions to this rule: finely chopped chives, fresh coriander, and parsley. Harvest with sharp scissors to avoid harming the stems, and chop with a sharp knife to preserve the oils in the leaves. Trim thyme and oregano after flowering to keep them tidy.

When to prune

Begin cutting back your oregano, rosemary, and thyme plants in the early fall. You can thin them out next spring by eliminating dead stems and stimulating new growth. In the fall, remove the leaves of chives, mint, and tarragon.

Care tips

Herbs can be protected under cloches when the season changes and they begin to lose their potency. Succulent herbs can be grown on sunny window sills all year round. Place pots on their feet in the winter to avoid waterlogging; keep them close to a wall for protection; and, if necessary, wrap them in insulation.

Choose your spot

As a general rule of thumb, it's recommended that you keep your herbs as close to your kitchen as possible so that they may be easily accessed when you're cooking. You can also plant herbs where you'll be entertaining or relaxing so you can enjoy the scent of their leaves.

Plan your garden plot, raised bed, or pots with these tips

When planning an herb garden, keep in mind that you need to be able to quickly gather the herbs you wish to use in your cooking. Using stepping stones to get to the herbs in the middle of a large plot is a good idea. Herb gardens that are round or oval can be walked around or through, while a triangle bed works well in the corner of a more miniature garden. Using bricks, bark chippings, or gravel, divide your herb garden into parts for herbs with similar growing requirements, like a cartwheel or checkerboard. It is possible to control the soil composition with a raised herb bed, allowing you to cultivate the plants you desire.

Another benefit is adding complexity to the garden and making harvesting easier. Place them in the middle of the bed for taller plants like bronze fennel. Try a variety of leaf shapes and colors, such as dark-leafed herbs next to golden-leafed ones – the contrast is stunning. Curly-leafed parsley and chives are excellent edging plants since they are easy to grow.

How to plant herbs

Well-drained soil is essential for most culinary herbs. Lightening the soil is necessary if the clay is too heavy. In regions where Mediterranean herbs will be grown, add horticultural grit to the soil by digging in some well-rotted compost. It would help if you used topsoil and horticultural grit from the garden center in a raised herb garden. Use an excellent, multipurpose compost in pots and add some horticultural grit or perlite for additional drainage. Before you plant the plants, you can ensure they're in the appropriate place. By researching its potential height and spread, you know how much room each herb will need to develop. Make sure to water well before planting.

How to care for your herb garden

Keep your new herb garden well-watered for the first several weeks, especially during the hottest months. As soon as you're halfway through your current batch of annual herbs, start a new one. When the weather is warm enough, sow seeds directly into the soil in a pot or tray of multipurpose compost. To give your perennials a boost, either remove some of the compost from their pots and repot them in fresh compost in the spring or repot them in new compost. In the second spring, divide chives, tarragon, and repot woody Mediterranean herbs like rosemary. During the fall, late autumn is the best time to remove herbs such as mint and chives from the garden. Pruning woody, evergreen herbs like rosemary and sage will keep them in shape after flowering or in the spring.

How to grow herbs

•Clove

After harvest, it is best to plant the clove seeds as soon as possible. They should be left in the flower bud to keep the seeds moist and viable until you can plant them. A wet, well-drained potting soil is ideal for sprouting clove seeds.

•Peppercorn

Vegetative cuttings are the most common method of propagation for black pepper vines, which are commonly interspersed amid shade trees like coffee. To grow black pepper plants, you need high temperatures, a lot of rain, and the soil that drains properly.

•Sage

To thrive, garden sage necessitates full light and well-drained soil. Perennial sages should be grown from seed, whereas annual and biennial sages can be started from seed. A wide variety of sages thrive in containers. You can trim down perennials after flowering, but leaves can be harvested whenever you need them.

•Rosemary

Rosemary thrives in broad light and well-drained soil. Before planting rosemary in the garden, it's best to cultivate it in containers for a few years to ensure that its roots aren't exposed to the elements in the winter. Then, to keep the plant from turning woody, cut it back every year and mulch it in the fall with leaf mold, well-rotted compost, or manure.

•Spirulina

Put the live spirulina culture in a transparent tank, add filtered water, and then add the Spirulina Nutrient Solution to the tank. You should maintain temperatures at 95°F in a warm, sunny location. Make sure the pH is between 8 and 10 by stirring the solution regularly. After 3 to 6 weeks, the crop is ready for picking.

•Dandelion root

Although dandelion plants enjoy full light, the most excellent greens are usually grown in partial shade. If you grow them in full sun, you can cover the plants with a box or a dark cloth a few days before harvesting to protect the foliage. The pH range of 6.2 to 6.8 is ideal for these taproot plants, which thrive in the slightly acidic soil found in lawns. If necessary, they can withstand a pH range of 6.0 to 8.5. When planting dandelions in poor soil, you can use compost to improve the quality of the soil.

• Peppermint

Although peppermint may thrive in a wide range of conditions, it favors a cool, damp climate and loose, organically rich soil. A pH of 5.5 to 6.0 is ideal for soil. It can grow in sandy or clay soil, as long as it's kept well watered. A perfect growing environment for peppermint is a site that receives direct sunlight for most of the day. Dry soil is a death sentence for any plant, regardless of the quality of the soil or the amount of sun it receives. But as harvest time gets closer, letting the soil dry out between waterings increases the amount of oil in it.

•Chamomile

You can start chamomile from seed or a live plant in spring. Growing chamomile from seed is more complicated than starting from plants or divisions, but it is still possible. Chamomile thrives in cool weather and prefers partial shade, although it can also thrive in full sun. The ground should be dry. Once your chamomile plant is well established, you won't have to do anything to maintain it. Chamomile thrives in a relaxed environment, as do the majority of herbs. However, many leaves with weak flavors and fewer blooms result from too much fertilizer.

●Milk thistle

For summer flowering, you should put the milk thistle seeds outside in either March or April, about 1/2 inch deep. You'll only need three or four seeds per hole if you drill your holes at a distance of three feet or more. Germination takes 10 to 20 days, during which you can thin out the weaker plants.

●Artichoke

Artichokes thrive in a warm sunny spot. To make optimal use of space, you should sow the seeds in a small pot and then transplant them into a bigger one. Since artichokes can thrive, you should plant them 60 cm apart. It would be best if you harvested them before they open and start to flower

●Slippery elm

It isn't difficult to develop slippery elm trees if you wish to do so. During the spring, harvest the sliding elm samaras. Depending on your preference, throw them from branches or sweep them from the ground. After air-drying the seeds for a few days, it's time to sow the slippery elm seeds.

●Marshmallow

Sow them in rows 18 to 24 inches apart, in clusters of five or six seeds. Keep them moist until they germinate by lightly covering them with soil. It usually takes between three and four weeks to complete this process. However, these resilient plants will come back year after year once they've been planted.

●Licorice root

Make your seed starting mix by following these recipe instructions and soaking the seeds for at least 24 hours in lukewarm water before planting. Then, at a depth of half an inch, plant the seeds. Keep the soil around the seeds moist until they sprout. Within two weeks, the seeds begin to grow. Germination occurs best at about 68 F. Each plant should have a 2-foot separation.

●Cinnamon

For the most part, gardeners do not start from seed. Give your cinnamon plants room to develop if you plan to cultivate them outside. You should plant apart from other trees and plants to get enough sunlight. Add compost to a hole twice the size of the root ball. Before you fill the planting hole with soil and carefully water it, ensure there are no air pockets.

●Elderberry

Plant elderberries at the same depth as their roots in the ground. Because elderberries have weak roots, it's essential to water them frequently during the first season. Apply irrigation if less than an inch of rain in a week to keep the soil moist but not soggy.

•Garlic

If you're planning to plant garlic, remember that it prefers well-drained, light soil in full sun. Break the bulbs into individual cloves and plant the larger ones with the flat end facing down and the pointy end 2.5 cm below the soil surface.

•Astragalus

Astragalus is more difficult to grow from seed than other herbs. Cold stratification of the seeds is required for at least three weeks. Soak or scarify the seed coat with fine-grade sandpaper before sowing to enhance germination. While it is possible to sow Astragalus herb plants in the garden directly, the standard recommendation is to start them indoors in late winter. Then, when the risk of frost has passed, transplant seedlings.

•Ginger

Before planting the ginger rhizome, split the ginger rhizome in half and allow the cut to heal and form a callus. Spring is the best time to plant rhizomes. The plant should fully develop the eyes on each piece as they grow. Good ginger plants are made from fresh rhizomes from another producer. The growth retardant in the ginger rhizome should be soaked

186

in water overnight. The rhizomes should be planted 2 to 4 inches deep, with the growing buds facing upward, six to eight inches apart.

●Echinacea

During the spring or fall, plant Echinacea plants in well-drained soil in full to partial sunlight. Echinacea can be grown from seed, but it needs a period of cold, damp stratification to germinate. To prevent birds from eating your seeds, scatter them widely in the fall (after a hard frost in the north and before winter rains elsewhere). In the spring, the seeds will sprout. One of the advantages of starting with transplants is that most plants will flower in their second year.

●Olive leaf

The Mediterranean environment is ideal for olives; as such, they do their best in settings that are as near to that as possible. Locate a location where you can get the maximum sun while still being protected by a brick wall; a south-facing area is ideal.

●Oregano

Make sure your oregano is in full bloom to get the most taste. If you're growing in a hot climate, provide some shade. Plant as soon as the danger of frost has passed in the spring. Others wait until later in the season to plant their seeds in hopes of a warm spring. The soil should be at least 70 degrees Fahrenheit.

●Ashwagandha

When planting ashwagandha seeds, ensure the soil temperature is around 70 degrees Fahrenheit. It will take two weeks for the seeds to grow. Keep the seedlings well-watered while they're getting their feet started. After a month of growth, remove the poorly grown plants and leave around 50 to 60 cm spacing between them.

●Rhodiola

The hardy perennial rose root, Rhodiola Rosea, is not frost-sensitive. Therefore, zone 1 is the most challenging place it can survive. A male and a female plant are needed to produce seeds for this plant, which is not self-fertile. Bees and insects pollinate plants. Rhodiola Rosea prefers full sun but will thrive in most soil types, even in locations where it is frequently subjected to drought. It may also withstand saline conditions.

●Tulsi

The best temperature for germination is between 60 and 70 degrees Fahrenheit. Sow the seeds indoors in a greenhouse or on a warm, sunny windowsill to get a head start on spring. To ensure good seed-to-soil contact, push down the tulsi seeds on top of the soil and cover them with a thin layer of compost or dirt. Next, spray the seeds with a watering can and plant them in a location that is both warm and shady. Keep the soil continually moist as soon as the seedlings begin to sprout.

•Ginseng

A depth of around 1 12 inches is recommended for seeds, while roots should be placed under 3 inches of soil in the spring and do best when planted in the early months of the season. Ginseng plants thrive in damp circumstances, yet they require minimal care. Plants should not be fertilized.

•Turmeric

The best time of year to start a garden is in the spring when the weather is warming up. First, select a place with loamy, organically rich soil drains well and receives full to partial sun. Plants that grow naturally in humid environments, such as those in tropical regions, are known as monsoon survivors. However, the soil must be able to drain properly, or the roots may rot out. Work the soil to a depth of 8 to 12 inches for best results. You can add compost to enrich it and enhance drainage if necessary.

•Reishi

Hardwood trees, including oak, elm, beech, and maple, are ideal for the growth of reishi. However, hemlock is the preferred conifer for several species. They prefer to grow near the base of trees or stumps, where they can be found in abundance. Higher-up tree bracket fungi are unlikely to be reishi. The ideal time to discover reishi in the wild is throughout the summer and fall. However, elder reishi can be found year-round on trees.

●Anise Seed

Anise thrives in soil with a pH of 6.3 to 7.0, which is somewhat alkaline. All-day sun and well-drained soil are required for anise plants. Remove all weeds, roots, and debris from the seed bed before sowing the seed. Until the plants are established, anise requires constant watering. After that, the plants can withstand periods of drought.

●Bloodroot

Bloodroot does best in moist, well-drained soil with a high concentration of organic matter. Moisture is critical throughout the growing season. That's where you'll find them if you look at where they're found in their native habitat. Humus-rich soils and pH levels of 5.5-7.6 are ideal.

●Camphor

Full sun or partial shade is ideal for the growth of camphor trees. Once established, camphor trees don't require as much watering as other trees, but watering is still necessary for the first few years after planting. So when you plant, don't think about moving it somewhere else in the future.

•Cedar

Plant cedar trees from spring to early fall in well-drained, healthy soil that you can find at your local garden centre. A wet, somewhat acidic soil is ideal for growing cedar. Depending on the variety of cedar, plants should be spaced between 3 and 5 feet apart. When planting, keep the plant's crown at least a few inches above the soil.

•Slippery Elm

The slippery elm tree prefers the moist, fertile soils typical of the orders Mollisol and Alfisol. Therefore, it is most likely to thrive in the humid, fertile soils of river terraces, streambanks, lower slopes, and bottomland. However, it is frequently found in relatively drier areas, particularly those of limestone origin.

•Eucalyptus

The best place to grow eucalyptus is in a warm section of the country, away from cold winds. For the first growing season, plant in the spring or early summer and provide regular irrigation. Then, if it's a shrub, thoroughly prune the entire thing in the spring.

•Fennel

Fennel thrives in soil that is rich in nutrients and quickly drains. You should add compost to the soil before planting.

When planting fennel, ensure it gets at least six hours of direct sunlight daily. Start your fennel seeds after the last spring frost. When young, this plant needs to be protected from light frosts, but it can endure them. Wrap it in a frost cloth.

•Rose

Any time of year is fine for containerized roses to be planted, but the beginning of autumn until the beginning of spring is ideal because this is the period of the year when they are dormant. Unfortunately, the frozen or damp ground makes planting your new hybrid tea rose impossible. You can keep plants in pots in an outbuilding that isn't heated, and bare-root roses can be "heeled in" by digging a trench in regular garden soil, putting the roots in it, covering them with soil, and pressing them down.

•Witch Hazel

Witch hazel plants are tolerant of a wide range of soil conditions. As an understory plant, they can flourish in full sun to partial shade. Except for frequent watering in the first season and pruning to shape as desired, witch hazel care is primary. A few browsing deer have little effect on the witch hazel, unaffected by harmful pests or diseases.

•Blackberry Leaf

Numerous plants are not required to produce fruit for blackberries and their hybrids, which are all self-fertile. Semi-erect cultivars should be spaced 5 to 6 feet apart. Relatively upright cultivars should be spaced three feet apart. 5 to 8 feet apart, trailing variety. Rows should be spaced 8 feet apart. One inch deeper than they were in the nursery, plant them.

•Plantain

It is essential to shield young plantain plants from wind and cold in the early stages of growth and provide them with well-drained soil and frequent irrigation. Ensure that the root ball is buried in a well-lit, well-ventilated area of your garden. Sow the plantain at the same depth as when it was in the pot. 4-6 feet is a good length for the plantain to have (1-2 m).

•Horsetail

Although You can transplant horsetail rhizomes, they are usually propagated from nursery plants rather than seeds. It would be best if you buried horsetail rhizomes at least 2 inches deep in the ground. The soil line should be level with the surrounding grade if you're using nursery-grown plants in pots. When the plants are young, it is essential to keep the soil moist. The plants can endure short periods of dry weather after they have grown accustomed to it.

•Yarrow

To stimulate compact development and a high number of blossoms, place the plant in a location that receives full sunlight. Yarrow is prone to lean growth in partial sunlight and shade. Well-drained soil is ideal for growing yarrow. It thrives in hot, dry circumstances; it will not tolerate soil that's always damp.

HARVESTING HERBS

Harvesting Herbs

The best time to gather an herb's oils is at their peak potency. The flavor and aroma of herbs are mainly due to the oils in the plant. A lot depends on the plant component you're harvesting and the purpose for which you will use it to determine the best time. A few popular rules of thumb to bear in mind are as follows:

• You can begin by harvesting the herb when it has a sufficient number of leaves to sustain itself. Up to 75% of the current season's crop can be harvested at once.

• As soon as the dew has evaporated in the morning, begin harvesting.

• You should collect herbs before blooming to ensure enough leaf output.

• Before the flowers have fully opened, you should harvest the buds of herbs to extract the maximum flavor and oil out of them.

• Just before they open is the ideal time for drying herbs.

• You can harvest up annual herbs to the first frost.

• Trimming perennial herbs in late August is an excellent idea. You should cease harvesting your crops about a month before the first frost. Pruning done too late can encourage growth that will not be able to withstand the winter chill.

• The second blooming season occurs in the fall when tarragon or lavender plants are sheared in half early in the summer.

How to harvest each part of the herb:

Leaves and aerial parts

The term "aerial" refers to sections of plants that grow above the ground's surface. At least two sets of leaves should remain on herbs with stems and leaves that branch off from the main stem for harvesting (most plants). More than one-third of the stem's length should be avoided during harvesting. The plant will look and recuperate better if you cut it just above a leaf node, where new growth is likely to develop. Chives and parsley, for example, don't branch or produce leaves; therefore, you'll cut the plant at its base.

Flowers and Buds

Pinch off the bud and any bracts connected to the flower's base while harvesting blooms or buds. Calendula, red clover, and chamomile, among other flowers, keep their full heads intact. However, if you like, you may just remove the petals (rose, dandelion). If you plan on drying flowers, consider using a dehydrator. When drying, place the flowers in a single layer. They will ferment and mold if you don't correctly dry the middles.

Bark

When the sap is increasing, and the trees have not yet leafed out in late fall or early spring, it is best to harvest the bark. It would be best if you did not cut off a live tree's bark. The initial phase is pruning twigs and branches up to 12 inches in diameter. Please remove any remaining leaves from the limbs once they have been cut. With a knife or peeler, remove the bark, and then use clippers to clean up the twigs after you're done. Make a tincture with 10% glycerin or honey if you intend to use the bark.

Roots

Like bark, roots are best collected in the spring or fall. Digging the roots may be as simple as loosening the soil around the plant with a garden fork. Using a sharp spade for root crowns or Hori Hori for slicing a portion off is excellent. You can remove the root with a digging stick or a CobraHead, but it will take more time and effort.

Herb Preservation

Drying, freezing, and culinary preservation are the most prevalent methods for preserving herbs.

Drying Herbs

After harvesting the herbs, thoroughly clean and dry them and remove any dead or damaged plants. The herbs should be tied loosely in bunches so that they may breathe. Put the bunches in little paper bags so the stems may be seen when the bags are opened. Vent the bag by opening the vents. During drying, the bags prevent the herbs from becoming contaminated. Next, place the herb bundles in a warm, dry place. The ideal location is a well-ventilated attic, garage, shed, or barn.

Tray drying

Tray drying is a suitable alternative for herbs with short stems or individual leaves. In a well-ventilated environment, lay the herbs on the tray in a single layer. The leaves may have to be rotated to guarantee a uniform drying process.

Drying with heat

You can dry herbs in a conventional oven, a microwave oven, or a dehydrating oven. Remove the leaves from the stems and store the dried herbs in an airtight container in a cool, dark location after drying. Avoid squeezing the leaves when picking herbs. Before using herbs in a dish, you should grind them to a fine powder. When properly preserved, most herbs retain their flavor for around a year. Cut the stems carrying the seed heads just before they turn brown if you want to dry the herb seeds. Place the stems in paper bags with holes punched in the sides and hang them upside-down. A warm, well-ventilated environment is essential while drying luggage.

Freezing

Fresh herbs can be harvested, washed, and chopped in addition to drying and freezing them in ice cube trays with water or oil. In a freezer-safe plastic bag, put the ice cubes. As needed, use individual cubes. Herb leaves can be blanched for a few seconds in boiling water and then cooled in ice water to preserve their flavor. You can then use plastic bags to store the leaves.

Culinary Preservation

Adding fresh herbs to olive oil, butter, or soft cheese before cooking is another way to preserve them for later use in meals. Kitchens are becoming increasingly familiar with herb-infused vinegar, which is rising in popularity. Preserve herbs and spices in your favorite cooking vinegar. To keep herbs fresh, store them with salt or sugar. As natural dehydrators, salt and sugar are excellent for preserving herbal specimens. Using a mason jar, put salt or sugar on the bottom and then stack the fresh herbs on top. To finish filling up the container, repeat Step 2. You can use herbs and flavored salt or sugar later.

PURCHASE YOUR HERBS

Herbal products

Traditional herbal products are frequently the most readily available. If you're looking for them, you can now find them on the internet and at your local grocery store. However, an individual or small business that makes the product on an as-needed basis should be questioned about the origins, preparation, and source of their herbs and how and why their dosage was determined. In addition, manufacturing and packaging may reduce the effectiveness of herbs in mass-produced. Fresh herbs that need to be shipped vast distances are likewise affected by this.

Purchasing herbs can be an alternative suitable for different situations. If the plant you want to grow does not grow appropriately within the conditions, you have in your region. It is recommendable to purchase it from a trustworthy shop. The reason for this lies in the product quality. Like humans, herbs can also be quite sensitive to their conditions; therefore, growing in non-suitable conditions may lead to a considerably less potent herb.

Also, consider the time each herb takes to harvest. Plants take time to grow and harvest, and their timing may clash with an urgent need for a specific herb. Consider purchasing a herb if you want a particular herb for the short term.

How do you locate herbalists?

The organizations listed here provide listings and directories for finding qualified herbalists.

●The National Certification Commission for Acupuncture and Oriental Medicine (NCCAOM)

●The National Ayurvedic Medical Association

●American Herbalists Guild

Herbal medicine has a wide range of certifications accessible. Expect little respect from your fellow herbalists if you are just starting out. Those who pursue advanced degrees in herbal medicine, such as a master's or a doctorate, must be licensed by their respective states. If you prefer to consult with a trained expert, NDs and acupuncturists are good choices. Some insurance plans may even cover visits to the doctor.

Online herbal stores

You can get high-quality herbs from these trusted online herbal retailers.

General herbal sources

- The San Francisco Herb Company

- Herbs of the Mountain Rose

- Five-flavor herbs

- Herb Store in Bulk

Ayurvedic herbal sources

- Banyan Botanicals

- The Ayurvedic Institute

Herbal sources for Chinese medicine

- Dandelion Botanicals

- Chinese Herbs Direct

A registered acupuncturist or Chinese herbalist is the only way to get a hold of Chinese herbal medication. Using the NCCAOM's directory of board-certified acupuncturists, you can find a practitioner in your area.

STEP THREE: USE YOUR HERBS IN THE BEST WAY

THE TOP 12 HERBS AND HOW TO USE THEM

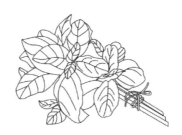

Basil

You can use it to make a classic pesto sauce, which goes well with fish or tomatoes. If you want to cook Italian-style,

208

look for sweet Genovese or Napoletano. If you're looking for something different, choose Greek, lettuce, or an aniseedy Thai dish.

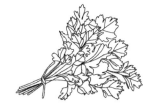

Parsley

This ingredient can be used to improve sauces, soups, stuffing, salad dressings, and garnishes. In addition, a cloche can extend the life of curly and flat-leaved kinds well into the fall and even into the winter if they have been correctly cared for.

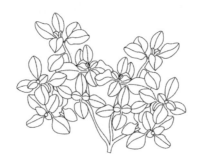

Lemon thyme

The foliage's versatility in the kitchen and its appeal to wildlife make it a popular ingredient. Potted plants of lemon and golden varieties are beautiful. For a delicate scent, plant creeping thyme in the cracks in the paving.

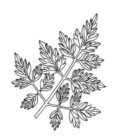

Chervil

Soups, sauces, egg dishes, and more benefit from its mild anise flavor. With its attractive foliage and fast seedling growth, curled chervil is a popular choice.

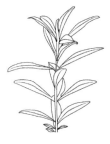

Tarragon

A staple in French cuisine and a must to improve a simple potato salad. French tarragon should be on your radar. Even though it's best to utilize the leaves immediately, they can be dried or stored in an airtight container until needed.

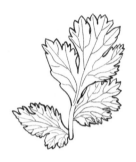

Coriander

Adding it to rice, couscous, and curries is a great idea. In addition, salads would benefit from the addition of flowers. Santos, a bolt-resistant cultivar of coriander, is a good choice because it doesn't go to seed as quickly.

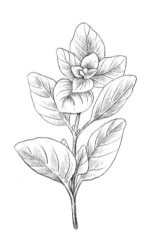

Oregano

Because it has a strong, pungent taste, it is often used dried instead of fresh in Italian, Greek, and Mexican cooking. Which dwarf varieties to look for include Kent Beauty, Common, and Compact Greek.

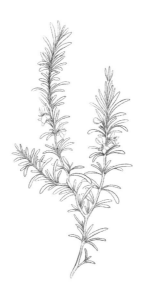

Rosemary

One of the favorite herbs when cooking lamb or pork dishes, giving an extra flavor that you are not going to regret. Most types can be used in the kitchen. Once planted in the ground, rosemary will continue to thrive for many years.

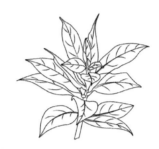

Bay Leaves

It's great in soups, stews, and mashed potatoes. The flavor of the leaves stays the same when they are dried, so this is an excellent way to do it. Look for hardier Angustifolia and Aurea types rather than the standard bay, which has dark, aromatic leaves.

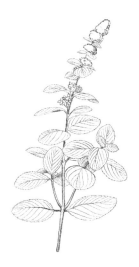

Mint

Tea, mojitos, and even mint sauce for meat can all benefit from a dash of this ingredient. Apple mint, English lamb mint, and spearmint are just a few common kinds (also known as garden mint).

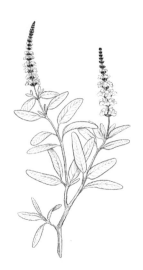

Sage

The savory sage-and-onion stuffing pairs wonderfully with the greens, giving it an extra flavor that gives life to the dish. The broad-leaved species of sage is an excellent alternative to common sage. If desired, grow from seed or cuttings.

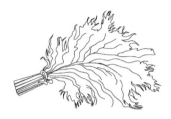

Dill

Treat them like bay leaves and let them flavor soups and stews. You can also add them to the cooking water while boiling potatoes. Dill seeds can be used whole or crushed, and they are frequently used in bread, soups, vegetable dishes, pickles and fish.

Seedlings or purchasing herb plants

Seed or plant? It all depends on what herbs you're using. Planting annuals like basil, dill, coriander, and parsley in pots or cell trays in the spring is the best way to ensure their long-term viability. Parsley is a tough biennial, whereas perennials like rosemary, thyme, oregano, and sage, which can live for several years, should be purchased as a plant. Summer is the best time to plant herbs as plugs because of the longer days and warmer soil. A couple of weeks should be enough time to reap the benefits of your hard work.

WAYS TO USE MEDICINAL HERBS AT HOME

7 Home Remedies Using Herbal Medicines

Herbal Tea: It is an excellent way to consume some herbs, especially for coughs and colds, because it may soothe an irritated throat as nothing else can. Echinacea, licorice root, ginger, lemon, and sage are a few of my favorite and most frequently recommended therapeutic plants for this technique. Use fresh or dried leaves, depending on your preference.

How to prepare herbal tea at home

Fresh leaves: Fresh herb leaves should be rinsed and placed in the bottom of a cup with around three large leaves. Take a cup of boiling water and pour it over the dish. Let it sit for up to seven minutes before serving.

Dried leaves: The best method is to use a tea ball or infuser with dried leaves. You can achieve your choice of strength by steeping the leaves in hot water for about seven minutes or until they have dissolved. At bedtime, a cup of chamomile tea is popular with many individuals.

Easy Mint Tea

- Prep time: 5 minutes

- Cook time: 1 minute

- Servings: 1

Ingredients

- Boiling water

- Fresh mint leaves – 8, left on the stem

Method

1. Place the mint in a mug and pour over the boiling water.

2. Steep for 5 minutes.

3. Enjoy.

Thyme Tea

- Prep time: 5 minutes

- Cook time: 1 minute

- Servings: 1

Ingredients

- Fresh thyme sprigs – 8

- Boiling water

Method

1. Place the thyme in a mug and fill the mug with boiling water.

2. Steep for 5 minutes and enjoy.

Lemon Ginger Tea

- Prep time: 5 minutes

- Cook time: 1 minute

- Servings: 1

Ingredients

- Grated fresh ginger – 1 tbsp.

- Boiling water – 1 cup

- Honey – 1 tbsp.

- Lemon juice – 1 tbsp.

Method

1. Place the ginger in a tea ball and then place it in a mug. Pour over the boiling water and steep for 5 minutes.

2. Remove the strainer. Stir in the lemon juice and honey and serve.

Flavoring options

Herbal Poultice: This is a method in which the plant's leaves (or roots, depending on the situation) are placed in a piece of gauze or muslin, applied to the affected area, and left on for the desired amount of time.

Herbal Poultice Preparation

To produce a poultice, you can either use raw leaves and roots or heat them.

For the **raw poultice**: Use a blender to make a puree of the leaves and roots, or chop them finely using a knife. Place the gauze or muslin over the top.

For a **hot poultice**: Put the leaves or roots in a pot with water that is two times the herb's volume. Bring 1/4 cup herbs and 1/2 cup water to a simmer and boil for a few minutes.

A poultice can be left on for as long as 24 hours, but a mustard poultice should only be put on for a few hours due to its hot-burning nature, while a comfrey poultice can be left on for as long as 12 hours. The length of time depends on the condition and the herb. Poultices should be changed regularly. To keep the poultice in place and protect your clothing, you'll need to cover it with gauze or breathable fabric.

Herbal Poultice

- Prep time: 5 minutes

- Cook time: 0 minutes

- Servings: 1

Ingredients

- Turmeric powder - 1 tsp.

- Chopped ginger - 1 ounce

- Raw sliced onion - ¼

- Garlic clove - 1 chopped

- Coconut oil - 2 tsp.

- Cheesecloth or cotton bandage

Method

1. Add everything to a pan and heat on low heat until dry.

2. Remove from the heat and cool to the touch.

3. Place the herb mixture on the center of the cloth and make a poultice.

4. Place on the affected area for 20 minutes.

Yarrow Poultice

- Prep time: 5 minutes

- Cook time: 0 minutes

- Servings: 1

Ingredients

- Fresh yarrow herb – 25 to 50g

- Water

Method

1. Add the herb and a bit of water to a blender and blend to make a paste.

2. Place the herb mixture on the center of a cloth and make a poultice.

3. Place on the affected area for 20 minutes.

Dried Herb Poultice

- Prep time: 5 minutes

- Cook time: 0 minutes

- Servings: 1

Ingredients

- A handful of dried herbs of your choice

- Boiled water

- Essential oils of your choice

Method

1. Add everything to a blender and blend to make a paste.

2. Place the herb mixture on the center of a cloth and make a poultice.

3. Place on the affected area for 20 minutes.

Infusion or Decoction

As a general rule, an herbal infusion is just a matured herbal tea. Allow the tea to steep for an hour instead of just a few minutes, resulting in a more robust cup of tea. A decoction is a hot water bath in which a smashed or chopped herb, root, or bark is allowed to boil and seep for an extended period.

The Hot Infusion Recipe

Method

1. Scoop 1 tbsp. Of dried herbs into a tea strainer. Then place it in a mug.

2. Add boiling water to cover.

3. Steep for up to 1 hour before straining.

Cold Infusion

Method

1. Place loose herbs in a jar.

2. Cap after filling with cold water.

3. Infuse overnight.

Decoctions

Method

1. In a pan, place 3 tbsp. Of dried herbs.

2. Cover the herbs with cold water.

3. Simmer, covered, for 20 to 45 minutes.

4. Strain, but do not discard the herbs.

5. Strain into a one-quart jar without discarding the herbs. Since some water will have evaporated, the liquid that has been filtered will not fill the jar.

6. Pour hotter (not boiling) water through the herbs in the strainer until the jar is full.

7. After the decoction is done simmering, you can add leafy herbs that can't handle a long-simmering time to the hot water. Then, after 10 to 15 minutes, you can filter the mixture again.

Syrup

For those with picky eaters or children, a syrup may be your best bet for getting them to take their medicine. Because medicinal syrups are shelf-stable and last longer than infusions or decoctions, you can prepare them in advance and have them ready to use when you're not feeling well. Make a decoction first, then add your sweetener to finish the syrup.

Elderberry Syrup

●

Prep time: 5 minutes

- Cook time: 10 minutes

- Servings: 1

Ingredients

- Dried elderberries - 3/4 cup

- Cinnamon stick – 1

- Whole cloves - 4-5

- Chopped ginger root - 1-2 teaspoons (fresh)

- Water - 4 cups

- Raw honey

Method

1. Combine everything in a pan. Cover partially and simmer until the liquid is reduced by half.

2. Strain and add honey. Store.

Ginger Syrup

- Prep time: 5 minutes

- Cook time: 10 minutes

- Servings: 1

Ingredients

- Grated ginger root - 1 cup

- Cinnamon chips – 1 tsp.

- Water – 4 cups

- Raw honey

Method

1. Combine everything in a pan. Cover partially and simmer until the liquid is reduced by half.

2. Strain and add honey. Store.

Throat and Cough Soothing Syrup

- Prep time: 5 minutes

- Cook time: 10 minutes

- Servings: 1

Ingredients

- Wild cherry bark - 2 tablespoons

- Rosehips - 2 tablespoons

- Mullein leaf - 1 tablespoon

- Licorice root - 1 tablespoon

- Elderberries - 1 tablespoon

- Cinnamon stick - 1

- Water - 4 cups

- Raw honey

Method

1. Combine everything in a pan. Cover partially and simmer until the liquid is reduced by half.

2. Strain and add honey. Store.

Tincture

Preparing a tincture is, in essence, the same as making an extract at home. Both alcohol and apple cider vinegar work, but alcohol has a longer shelf life and is less likely to mold. Taken alone, tinctures can be added to syrups and salves and can even be used as an ingredient in lotions.

Tincture Recipe

Method

1. Fill 1/3 of a glass jar with chopped fresh leaves.

2. Fill half the jar with berries, bark, roots, or dry leaves.

3. Then fill 2/3 of the jar with berries, bark, or roots.

4. Pour alcohol (70%) over the herbs and cover completely.

5. Cover the jar with parchment paper.

6. Then cover with a lid.

7. Allow sitting for 6 to 8 minutes.

8. Strain and store the tincture.

Burdock Root

1. Chop several fresh herbs and put them in a glass container.

2. Fill the jar with vodka (50% alcohol).cover and set aside for two weeks.

3. Strain and store.

Basic Herbal Tincture

- Fresh herbs - 1 ounce, chopped fine

- 100-proof vodka - 3 ounces

Or

- Dried herbs - 1 ounce

- 100 proof vodka - 5 ounces

Method

1. Place herbs in a jar and pour in the vodka. Cover the herbs.

2. Cover the jar and place it in a cool, dry place for two weeks.

3. Shake the jar regularly.

4. Strain and store.

Salves, balms, creams, and lotions

You can add essential oils and other medicinal herbs to many homemade skincare products, such as ointments and balms. This is typically accomplished by the use of herbal infusions in your oil. This is a straightforward technique, but it does require some forethought. You can use herbs to infuse the oil. Place the jar on a sunny ledge and shake it every few days as it seeps for 6 to 8 weeks. Use the infused oil in your favorite recipe once it has steeped for eight weeks.

Herbal Salve

- Infused herbal oil - 8 oz.

- Beeswax -1 oz. either grated or pellets

Method

1. Warm the oil and the melted beeswax.

2. Mix well and pour into containers.

3. Put the cap and store it.

Soothing Herbal Balm

- Herbal oil infusion - 4 oz.

- Olive oil - ¾ cup

- Beeswax - 3 tbsp.

Method

1. On low heat, melt the beeswax and add the oil.

2. Add the herbal oil infusion. Mix and store.

Lotion Recipe

- Infused avocado oil - 1 tbsp.

- Avocado butter - 1 tbsp.

- Emulsifying wax - 1 tbsp.

- Distilled water - 6 tbsp.

- Preservative of choice

Method

1. Combine wax, butter, and oil in a jar.

2. Heat the jar over indirect heat.

3. Stir and cool. Repeat for several minutes.

4. Remove from the heat and add the preservative.

5. Store.

Herbal Steams

Herbal steam not only freshens the air in your home but also provides medicinal effects. For congestion, peppermint and eucalyptus are popular choices. However, people prone to seizures should exercise caution when using either, and you should use neither peppermint nor eucalyptus with children younger than six years old. Allow the herbs to boil in water for a few minutes before serving. Alternatively, place the herbs in a heat-resistant bowl and cover with just simmering water.

Decongesting Herbal Steam

Ingredients

- Eucalyptus leaves - ¼ cup

- Peppermint leaf - 2 tbsp.

- Rosemary leaf - 2 tbsp.

- Thyme - 3 tbsp.

- Lavender buts - 1 tbsp.

- Sea salt - ¼ cup

Method

1. Mix all of the herbs and salt. Pour in a jar.

2. Boil water and add 1 tbsp. Of the herbal salt mixture.

3. Pour boiling water over the herbs and cover the bowl. Steep for 5 to 10 minutes.

4. Position your face over the bowl and cover your head with a towel.

5. Inhale the steam for 10 minutes or more.

HERBAL MEDICINE SAFETY TIPS

You can avoid a potentially harmful reaction to herbal medicines if you follow these top tips:

Do your homework

It's easy to get sucked into the latest fads and fill your shopping basket with everything that sounds promising. When it comes to food, however, you'd better have an idea of what you're about to put in your mouth. Herbal supplements are no different, except that they are much more potent. With blueberries, you can naturally improve your eyes. Black cohosh may also help balance hormones. Consider the supplement's possible advantages and potential hazards and side effects before making a decision (an herbal guide like this is an excellent place to start). Another option is to speak with a herbalist or naturopathic physician who has received specialized training and will put your health and well-being first. It's a no-brainer to take the time and effort commitment when it comes to your health.

Check for a seal of approval

The components and concentrations of the various brands are different. You should thoroughly inspect the labels of the natural herbs you are considering once you have narrowed your options. The first important thing to look for is if the herb is standardized, a process in which the active ingredients of the plant are chemically analyzed. The FDA's Current Good Manufacturing Practices (CGMP) certify that manufacturing processes are up to current standards and substantiate the product's strength, quality, purity, and identity while screening for contaminants, deviations, mix-ups, and other errors. Check the label to make sure the supplement meets these criteria as well. What if you come upon a component that you think is suspicious? Consult your doctor or a herbalist if you have any concerns. In the end, it's better to be overprotective regarding your health.

Take your condition into account

Barley, hops, marijuana, and poppies come from nature, as do herbal supplements. In other words, consider your current health status before making a purchase, much less consuming something. Have a baby on the way? Learn about the potential side effects of herbal supplements on your child. You may want to see your doctor if you have a heart issue or allergies. You should take any medication with the same caution. When it comes to herbal supplements, the more you know about their effects on the body, the better equipped you will be to protect yourself.

Do your research on possible drug interactions before using any herbal supplements

When used with some pharmaceuticals (as well as certain meals and beverages like alcohol), herbal supplements can adversely influence the way other chemicals are digested, increasing the side effects of some medications while reducing their therapeutic benefits. Consult with your pharmacist or doctor before taking any medication.

You are aware of the source

According to recent studies, some herbal supplements imported from other nations may not be what they claim to be or may have been cultivated with pesticides and other toxins. In addition, the presence of heavy metals such as cadmium, lead, mercury, and others in other imported goods raises the possibility of health problems. Therefore, knowing where your supplement comes from is critical to its safety and efficacy. Can you trust the company that makes it? What country is the herbal supplement made in? What environment did it go through during the growing and processing stages? How and at what time should I be concerned? You'll be safer and closer to ideal health if you learn more about the ingredients in your herbal supplements and avoid any potentially harmful or false promises.

Preserve herbs in a cool, dry place

Keep your herbs fresh, safe, and flavorful with these tips.

● To avoid food poisoning, only buy fresh herbs that have been washed and are free of any dirt or other contaminants. Remove and discard any wilting stems or leaves at home.

● Keep them cool. Fresh herbs should be refrigerated as soon as you arrive home from the market, much like other perishable goods.

● Keep them in a safe place. Most herbs can be stored in a plastic bag in your refrigerator for up to five days without being washed. A plastic bag wrapped loosely over the leaves of herbs like basil and cilantro will keep them fresher for longer if kept in a glass of water.

• Cleanliness is essential. Use warm soapy water to clean your hands before handling fresh plants thoroughly. Then, wash and dry your herbs with a clean paper towel after they have been washed in cold water. Use a cutting board made just for fruits and vegetables to avoid bacteria from raw meat, poultry, or shellfish.

• Make sure to include dried herbs in your shopping list. Herbs can be safeguarded by storing them in a pantry or a locked cabinet. They can be kept in an airtight container for up to two years.

Herbs fresh from the garden and food sickness are linked

It's possible to get sick from eating fresh herbs because they are grown close to the ground and exposed to dirt. In addition, you may become ill if you eat fresh herbs that dangerous bacteria have tainted. Food sickness caused by Cyclospora and E. coli has been connected to the use of tainted plants.

In the field, fresh herbs can be affected by:

• Soil

• Animals

- Contaminated water

- Improperly composted manure

They are also susceptible to bacterial contamination:

- Harvest to post-harvest storage to transportation.

- Through cross-contamination with hazardous bacteria from raw meat, poultry, or shellfish at the grocery store, refrigerator, or cutting board.

Choosing herbs

- Look for fresh-smelling herbs with vibrant leaves. The stalks and leaves should be crisp but not dried out.

- Avoid leaves that are turning yellow or brown or have black patches.

Chilling/storing

- It is best to keep fresh herbs in the refrigerator unwashed. A plastic bag with an airtight seal is all that is needed. You can keep fresh herbs in the crisper or vegetable bin in your refrigerator for up to five days.

- After washing and drying with paper towels, you can put fresh herbs in freezer bags and put them in the freezer.

• Before cooking with basil, it should not be rinsed, dried, or chilled. This may turn the basil leaves black if you refrigerate them.

• This is the only procedure that should be utilized when dealing with herbs.

Cleaning

• Food poisoning can spread if you don't wash your hands and use proper cleaning methods.

• Clean all utensils, countertops, and cutting boards with soap and warm water before and after using fresh herbs.

Preparing

Make sure you wash your hands for at least 20 seconds with soap and warm water before and after you work with fresh herbs.

• You should throw yellowing or black patches on leaves away.

• Use cool running water to clean fresh herbs thoroughly. When it comes to washing herbs, nothing but water will do. Using cleaners is just as effective as gently washing them with water.

● You should not soak fresh herbs in a sink of water. There is a risk that they will become infected with bacteria from the sink.

CONCLUSION

A whopping 80 percent of the world's population relies on herbal medical items and supplements for some of their fundamental healthcare needs. The efficacy of a wide variety of herbal drugs has been successfully proved in therapy employing these components. People in many different countries are adopting herbal medications and other types of nutrients, or "nutraceuticals," to help them with a wide range of health concerns. Over the last few decades, herbal remedies have become more common in pharmacies and grocery stores, which shows that people are more interested in natural remedies.

As a prominent part of many countries' cultures, traditional herbal therapy is an essential component for many of the world's people. As a result, the amount of money spent on herbal products by people who use them at home or buy them over the counter is billions of dollars. Because of this, herbal remedies are typically considered a moderate and balanced way to heal. This helps explain why sales of herbal medicines are on the rise and now account for a significant portion of the global pharmaceutical market.

There are several scenarios in which herbs can be a lifesaver. It was standard practice to employ herbal remedies for health and well-being before the development of modern medicine. However, things took a turn for the worse after the introduction of modern synthetic medications. Making modern medicine and health care a business has made the pharmaceutical industry a fortune. Because of this, more and more people are turning to traditional therapy, which focuses on treating symptoms instead of the problems themselves.

After reading this book, you will no longer rely on conventional treatment to become a healthier person. So, what are you waiting for? Herbal treatments do not necessitate a steep learning curve. Some of the most commonly used herbs can be purchased or gathered to be used in recipes or to create remedies.

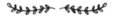

Special Offer

As part of the book, it is included a completely FREE Bonus guide that includes simple and surprising hacks and tips to improve your cooking skills. If you want to discover the 7 Fascinating Hacks and Tips for cooking with herbs, click on the link or scan the QR code below.

Link

https://mailchi.mp/a0e0be324cea/7-fascinating-hacks-and -tips-for-cooking-with-herbs

QR Code

Printed in Great Britain
by Amazon

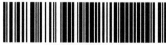

15793676R00147